CU00836296

The BMA Family Doctor Guide

Menopause

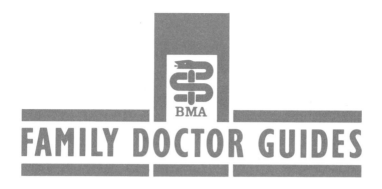

Menopause
Treating the symptoms

Mr Peter Bromwich, MRCOG

Series editor: Dr Tony Smith

Mr Bromwich is gynaecologist at Little Aston Hospital, Sutton Coldfield.

Published by Equation in association with the British Medical Association

First published 1989

© British Medical Association 1989

British Library Cataloguing in Publication Data

Bromwich, Peter
  Menopause.
  1. Women. Menopause
  I. Title II. Series
  612'.665

  ISBN 1-85336-051-1

Picture acknowledgements
John Rae: p. 17, 23, 27, 32, 35, 75, 79; Family Planning Association: p. 30; BUPA: p. 85, 89; Raymond Fishwick: cartoons; David Woodroffe: diagrams.

Equation, Wellingborough, Northamptonshire NN8 2RQ, England

Typeset by Columns of Reading
Printed and bound in Great Britain by The Bath Press, Avon.

10 9 8 7 6 5 4 3 2 1

Contents

1 Introduction

The menopause shares much with pregnancy. Both are significant landmarks in a woman's life, when profound hormonal changes interact with emotional events that go alongside important social changes in her role and the structure of her family. In both pregnancy and the menopause some of the problems that matter most to many women, and cause them the most concern, have not been studied by doctors in nearly the depth that they merit. Some women say that they have heard the same homily at different times from their doctors: 'Don't worry, it's only your age/because you are pregnant. It'll get better when you get used to it. Just give it time.' Many women who are going through the menopause feel very alone and have no one to talk to or turn to for advice. Their anxieties may be compounded by the fact that there are many myths about the menopause, and not all of these are old wives' tales either – the medical profession itself has been responsible for some of them.

The invisible menopause

Why is there so little knowledge about something so important that affects so many people? Some women feel that if the menopause affected men, a great deal more research would have gone into it! One reason might be that since the menopause is an inevitable stage in a woman's life, some doctors and other medical opinion-makers feel that its investigation and treatment is as unnecessary as that of a young girl's first period. Furthermore, their medical training emphasises this, as the menopause is ignored in many medical school curricula. And because the menopause is so common it does not interest medical researchers as much as something more rare. There is even no agreement on the symptoms that are associated with the menopause. Just as no two doctors will have the same view of the importance and relevance of the menopause to modern medicine so no two women will experience the same set of symptoms or, if they do, they may not attribute them to the menopause.

7

Why is a 'natural' event regarded as a new phenomenon?

In the past most people believed that men and women could only live for 'three score years and ten', after which their useful life was over. Even then, few lived until they were 70. Most died much younger than this and the average person could expect to live for only 40 or 50 years. Much has changed – not only do most of us live beyond our biblical span, but we are expected to work and fend for ourselves for nearly all of that time. It is not that humans have somehow managed to achieve a longer lifespan, but rather that many more of us are reaching our full allotment. You will see from the graph that average life expectancy has only recently begun to exceed the average age of the menopause; this explains in part why the menopause has come to be seen as a 'new' or 'unnatural' phenomenon that did not bother us three generations ago. Once, most women would have died before they needed to worry about the menopause.

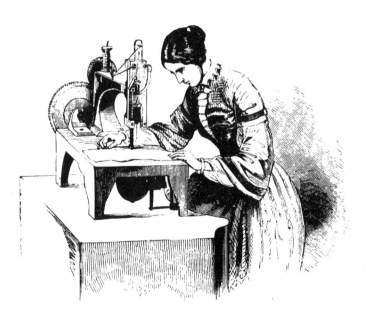

In the past many women died before they had to worry about the menopause.

Understanding helps

This book provides an honest view of the menopause, and the ways of alleviating some of its more troublesome symptoms. It discusses current thinking on the prevention of a condition called osteoporosis (the weakening of bones) that was once considered the inevitable consequence of ageing in women. It describes the more common attitudes and approaches to the menopause and the role of treatment. The menopause is not a disease and so it does not need treatment, but some of the symptoms associated with it can be helped, not necessarily by drugs. For many women the worst thing about the menopause is the fear of the unknown – reading this book should remove much of that fear.

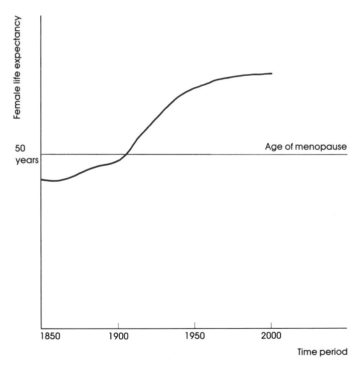

Relationship between life expectancy and average age of the menopause.

2 What happens at the menopause

'Menopause' means the end of menstruation, and it is simply the last of the approximately 400 periods a woman has. Periods stop when the ovaries no longer mature eggs in response to the hormone signals that reach them from the pituitary (a gland at the base of the brain that produces several important hormones).

About hormones

Hormones are chemical messengers that are released by glands directly into the blood stream, to be carried around the body. They may act on one organ only or they can affect the whole body. The pituitary gland produces hormones that usually act on other glands that in turn produce hormones that are able to act on the whole body. Thyroid stimulating hormone, for example, comes from the pituitary and acts on the thyroid gland to make it produce thyroxine, a hormone that acts on almost every cell in the body. The pituitary produces two hormones, follicle stimulating hormone and luteinising hormone, which act on the ovaries. 'Sex hormones' is a fairly sloppy form of medical shorthand for the hormones produced principally by the sexual organs (the ovaries and testes). These hormones can also be produced elsewhere in the body, however, mainly as a by-product of other processes.

The menstrual cycle

The menopause, like the start of menstruation, is triggered by hormonal changes in the body. It will probably help you to understand what happens during the menopause if we look at the menstrual cycle first.

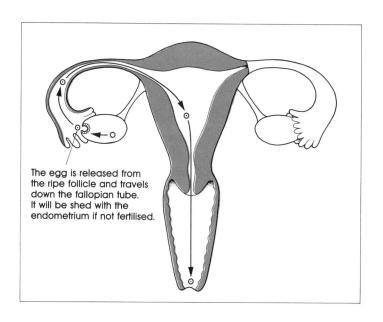

The egg is released from the ripe follicle and travels down the fallopian tube. It will be shed with the endometrium if not fertilised.

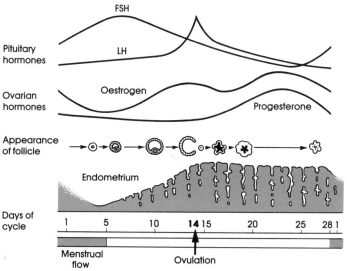

What happens during the menstrual cycle.

A typical cycle

A typical menstrual cycle takes about 28 days (although this can vary between women). The first day of bleeding is usually counted as day 1.

Days 1–5

Falling levels of the hormone progesterone in the body trigger the beginning of menstruation – the shedding of the lining of the womb together with a little blood. At the same time, follicle stimulating hormone and luteinising hormone, produced by the pituitary, stimulate the ripening of an egg in the ovary. This in turn produces increasing levels of oestrogen.

Days 5–14

Bleeding usually stops by day 5. Between days 9 and 13, the levels of oestrogen reach their peak. On day 13 the levels of follicle stimulating hormone and luteinising hormone reach their peak and ovulation takes place on day 14.

Days 15–28

If the egg is not fertilised, the level of oestrogen drops appreciably and the follicle from which the egg was released forms into a gland called the corpus luteum, which produces progesterone.

Days 24–28

The corpus luteum begins to degenerate and progesterone levels begin to fall. Some women begin to notice premenstrual symptoms such as breast tenderness and mood changes and they may also feel slightly bloated because of fluid retention. On day 1 bleeding begins again.

The ovary

The ovary does not have the ability to make new eggs throughout life; egg production fails once a woman has used all of the eggs she was born with. The graph shows the usage of eggs (oocytes) throughout life. As we have seen, eggs are not the only things the ovary produces and much of this book is about the effects on the rest of the body of the hormones produced by the ovary – the female sex hormones the oestrogens and the progesterones.

Oestrogens and progesterones

Oestrogens are produced constantly, but in varying amounts, and not only from the ovary, while progesterone is produced principally in the second half of the menstrual cycle. Oestrogens are responsible for most of a woman's sexual characteristics, while progesterone prepares her body for pregnancy. The cells that surround and are in close contact with the egg produce most of the female sex hormones, but although these cells are still present after the menopause, they do not seem to produce hormones if there is no egg to be developed.

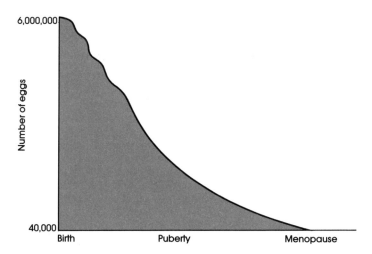

Women are born with a large number of eggs that are gradually used up.

Hormone levels at the menopause

When eggs are not produced the ovaries no longer secrete sex hormones on a regular cyclical basis (but some still come from other parts of the body). This lack of hormones leads to most of the problems that surround the menopause or develop after it.

The climacteric

Strictly speaking those years before and after the last period are known as the climacteric, and the menopause is simply the last period itself. 'Climacteric' comes from the Greek words for 'a step on a ladder', because it represents the beginning of the next phase in a woman's life. For most women, however, the terms climacteric and menopause are synonymous with 'the change'.

> **Most of the problems that surround the menopause or develop afterwards are caused by a lack of hormones.**

When does the menopause begin?

For most women their last period comes between their 50th and 51st birthday, with the climacteric beginning some years before and continuing for a few years afterwards. The graph shows the distribution of ages at which the menopause occurs in a large sample of women; as you can see quite a range of ages is possible.

The menopause occurs at a similar age in mothers and daughters, and a woman is likely to have her menopause at the same age as her sisters. Obviously periods stop immediately after a hysterectomy (the surgical removal of the uterus or womb), but even if the surgeon leaves the ovaries alone, symptoms of the menopause occur at a younger age in women who have had a hysterectomy. This suggests that some incidental damage happens at the time of surgery. The menopause occurs about a year earlier than average in women who smoke cigarettes, and up to a year later in women blind from birth. Going on the birth control pill for many years does not seem to affect the age at which the menopause happens, despite the fact that the combined pill prevents the release of eggs for all the years that a woman takes it. Eggs that are not released do not seem to be saved, and neither does the pill seem to affect in any way the quality or the number of those eggs left behind.

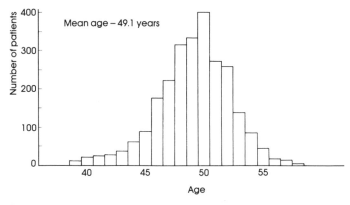

Distribution of ages at which menopause occurs.

Hormonal changes after 40

From the age of 40 your ovary becomes less responsive to the pituitary hormones that control it. The effect of this is to make you less fertile, to reduce the amounts of ovarian hormones you produce, and to alter the relative amounts of oestrogen and progesterone produced. There is also a change in the proportion of the different oestrogens produced.

Effect on the premenstrual syndrome

A change in the ratio between the hormones oestrogen and progesterone is responsible for the premenstrual syndrome. Some women find that the syndrome gets worse during the years of the climacteric and others that they get it for the first time, but in all women the menopause is the end of it. In a failing ovary the delicate balance between the two sets of hormones, oestrogen and progesterone, is lost as hormone production declines, producing an effect on the premenstrual syndrome as well as the periods.

Effect on periods

The endometrium will be scanty (if there is little oestrogen to make it grow in the first place) or irregular and less well organised (which usually means thicker or more overgrown) if oestrogen is produced in the first two weeks after menstruation, but is not followed by enough progesterone to organise the endometrium. When the endometrium is scanty, periods are light or may even be missed but when it is thick periods are usually heavy, may be long, are often irregular, and sometimes there is bleeding at odd times of the month as pieces of 'loose' endometrium are shed by the body.

Determining hormone changes

Measuring these hormone changes can confirm that the climacteric has started. Estimating the levels of oestrogen in the blood is of little relevance because they vary so widely throughout the month. It is much more useful to measure the blood levels of follicle stimulating hormone. Follicle stimulating hormone, you will remember, is the pituitary hormone responsible for making ovarian follicles grow. When the ovaries stop responding to the pituitary, the body reacts at first by increasing the amount of follicle stimulating hormone it produces, to try and stimulate the flagging ovary. This means that levels of follicle stimulating hormone rise in the blood, and so, if they are found to be high the implication is that the ovary is failing.

Considerations and implications

There are several important points for you to consider at the time of the menopause. Although your fertility is reduced, pregnancy can still occur, and because periods are often irregular there can be either a false reassurance that pregnancy is unlikely or has not occurred, or increased anxiety that it might have happened. Contraceptive needs are not constant throughout life, and methods suitable earlier on may be less appropriate now. Gynaecological problems may become obvious for the first time and can also change contraceptive suitability. Contraceptive methods are covered in the next chapter, but in general you will need to continue using something until you have had no periods for at least one year. If you are having the symptoms of the climacteric, your blood levels of follicle stimulating hormone are high, and you have had no periods for six months, however, you probably need not worry about conceiving.

Relief and regret

For most women the fact that fertility (and menstruation) are ending soon is a boon. For those who are childless, however, especially if it has not been through choice, the menopause can be an especially depressing time.

Liberation

The late 40's and the early 50's are an important time for women who are building careers. Changing careers becomes difficult later because most employers are unwilling to accept the challenge of retraining someone who may only be able to work with them for a decade or so before retiring. Good employers leap at the opportunity given them by a new employee with a wide background of experience capable of being able to devote time and energy without the potential distractions of pregnancy. This is one of the many reasons that some women say the menopause is liberating for them.

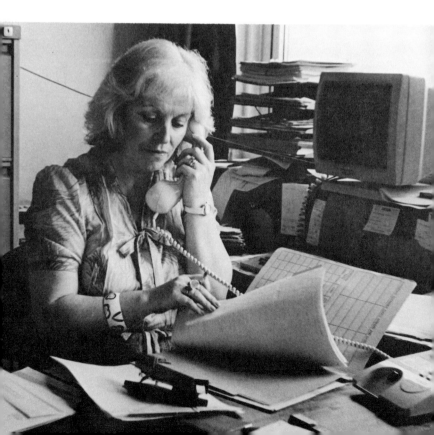

Heart disease

From a medical point of view the two most important changes to occur at the menopause are the increased likelihood of heart and blood vessel disease and the loss of mineral and protein that occurs in the bones (osteoporosis). Each of these problems has a chapter in its own right. Before the menopause women are relatively well protected against heart attacks and strokes – among those who do not smoke these are extremely rare. This protection is lost after the menopause, however, and 20 years later, heart attacks and other forms of blood vessel disease are as common among women as they are among men of the same age. Twenty years may seem a long time for all protection to go, but since rates in men are actually increasing all that time the rates for women have to accelerate just to catch up.

Osteoporosis

Before the menopause women have much more resilient bones than they do after it; this resilience is gradually lost over the rest of their life. Old people are much more likely to suffer from broken bones than the young; even children who are active and expose themselves to risks in sport and at play are not as likely to suffer serious bone fractures as older people. There are several important reasons for this, but the most important is the development of osteoporosis, the weakening of bone after the loss of protein and minerals, particularly calcium. The prevention of osteoporosis arouses controversy, but the long term nature of the changes in bones means that the definitive studies are unlikely to be finished this century. Osteoporosis is discussed in chapter 4.

3 The effects of the climacteric

Hundreds of symptoms are said to be associated with the climacteric, and perhaps three quarters of all women will have at least one of them as they reach or pass the menopause. Unfortunately, quite a few are not related to the level of hormones produced by the ovaries and one of the many things that has bedevilled people concerned about the menopause is the way all sorts of odd symptoms and complaints are blamed on the menopause, rather than being investigated and treated properly. Even the symptoms caused by oestrogen deficiency affect different women in different ways and to different degrees. Just as no two people who share similar life experiences will have the same feelings about them, so no two women will have the same attitude to the climacteric. The most important points that determine a woman's view are how emotionally prepared she is for the climacteric and her oestrogen hormone levels.

Oestrogen and weight

Oestrogens are secreted by the ovary, and their production declines in the years before the last period. Despite this the ovary continues to produce some hormones for several years after the menopause. Similar hormones are also produced by the adrenal glands (two small glands that sit just above the kidney), and these hormones are changed elsewhere in the body, principally by fat cells, to more active female sex hormones. Since fat women can do more of this than thin ones, fat women tend to have more female hormones in their blood than thin ones. To see how fat or thin you are use the formula overleaf to establish your 'Quetelet index'. Most people in the normal healthy range have a Quetelet index of between 20 and 25; if you have a value less than 20 you may be underweight while an index greater than 25 suggests that you are overweight!

$$\text{Quetelet Index (QI)} = \frac{\text{body weight (kg)}}{\text{height (m) x height (m)}}$$

So if you weigh 65 kg and are 1.7 m tall your index will be 22 which is in the normal health range.

Hot flushes

The commonest symptom of the menopause is also the hardest to describe. Like many things in life, if you need to have it described to you you have never had one. The hot flush (called the hot flash in the United States, which is perhaps a better term) is a sudden feeling of intense heat, that starts in the upper body and spreads over the face, and sometimes over the rest of the body. It is an unpleasant sensation, embarrassing as well as uncomfortable. Women who have it say that it feels as if a wave of fire is passing through them, and not only is it uncomfortable but the thought that they are behaving strangely while in company can be upsetting socially, perhaps leading to a loss of confidence or a wish to avoid potentially embarrassing situations like parties. Like many upsetting things, hot flushes are more obvious to the woman who has them than to the people around her. Eating hot or spiced food or drinking alcohol often provokes hot flushes. Many women want to run outside into cool air when having one, and so they begin to avoid eating in company or in restaurants.

Not a neurotic symptom

Because the effect is most noted by the woman who has the flush, it was once thought to be largely a neurotic symptom and always exaggerated. This is wrong – flushes are real sensations and are caused by changes in the sensitivity of small blood vessels in the skin, and the nerves that control them. Nobody knows exactly how they are caused but they are related to the levels of oestrogen in the blood. When these levels become very low, as they do some years after the menopause, flushes stop. Flushes occur when the body mistakenly thinks that you are very hot and so diverts blood from the inside to your skin. This is a normal body mechanism for cooling down someone who is hot, and sensitive equipment has shown that during a flush the temperature of a woman's skin rises by 5°C, while the temperature of the inner body falls by 0.5°C.

Coping with flushes

Raising the amount of oestrogens in your body will help get rid of flushes but so will learning to cope with them. Avoid tight clothes and things that constrict the neck, such as scarves or collars. Wearing several layers of thin clothing so that you can take off a layer, if necessary, is also sensible. If hot or spicy food provokes flushes, then be careful with your diet. Have a tepid shower (if it is possible) when you are feeling uncomfortably hot.

> **Spicy foods, alcohol, tea, coffee and some drugs can make hot flushes worse.**

Night sweats

The next characteristic symptom is night sweating – you wake up drenched in sweat. This is not just a little perspiration after hot flushes during sleep, it is really heavy sweating, that means you may have to change the bed clothes during the night. Not surprisingly, night sweating not only interferes with your sleep but also with your partner's. You both end up tired and irritable after a few weeks of sleepless nights. Night sweats are also caused by the changes that falling oestrogen levels produce in blood vessels and in their control.

Sleeplessness

Insomnia is common at the time of the menopause, but this may be related to the tensions produced by night sweats, hot flushes, and the other changes. Palpitations may also occur and the heart rate increases by as much as 20%.

Mouth changes

Teeth and mouth changes happen too. For some women this is no more than a transient problem when their mouth tastes coppery. This passes, although women who depend on their palate for their living, such as wine tasters or chefs, sometimes say that they lose fine discrimination. Other women develop gum problems, and sometimes teeth become looser, particularly if bone is lost from the jaws.

Skin irritability

Some women suffer from formication, a sensation of irritability under the skin rather like that of ants eating away. In fact the name comes from 'formica' the Latin for ant. It is difficult to control and seems to be quite separate from other skin signs of falling oestrogen levels.

These symptoms respond to oestrogen

All of these changes will eventually get better if left alone, but in 25% of women they will take up to five years to settle of their own accord. This is a long time to suffer, but unfortunately the unpredictable nature of these symptoms makes it difficult to say for how long treatment aimed at easing them should continue. All these symptoms, however, will respond to oestrogen replacement which we will discuss in chapter 8.

Psychological changes

Other changes also occur at the menopause. Harder to measure, but as important, are the psychological changes. These may result indirectly from the physical disturbances, but are probably caused directly by the altered hormone levels. Irritability and mood swings are common, but much more important are the attacks of anxiety, loss of memory, and loss of concentration. All of these will interfere with social and business life, and all may feed on each other to become bigger and bigger problems.

Depression may occur for the first time in some women. Sometimes depression is a normal response to the social and physical changes that are often experienced at this time of life, but some women develop an inner or 'endogenous' depression that is out of proportion to their personal circumstances and may be difficult to shift. Depression is often helped by giving replacement oestrogen hormones.

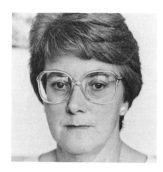

Anxiety and depression are not uncommon at this time.

Long-term effects of oestrogen loss

Many of the more obvious symptoms associated with the menopause are linked to the loss of oestrogen from the ovary, which acts particularly on the genital tissues but also affects almost every other cell in the body. The acute or abrupt effects have already been described but there are also long term effects. Oestrogens are important as 'anabolic' hormones; this means that for those cells that are sensitive to them and contain receptors (specialised parts of the cell wall that respond to oestrogens) they control the way cells grow and make tissues more complex and stronger. Tissue loss is the most important physical effect of a lack of oestrogen. Tissue loss in the vagina means that there is shrinking, loss of sensation as nerves decay, and loss of muscle. The lining of the vagina becomes weaker and less able to resist damage and so intercourse becomes more painful and more likely to result in bleeding.

Loss of libido

For many women the menopause is accompanied by a loss of libido, or sexual drive. There is one obvious physical cause for this—if the only sensation intercourse gives is pain then the want for it will decline. There is also a hormonal basis for the loss of libido in some women, because replacement of normal levels of ovarian hormones often leads to a return of sexual feelings.

For some women the loss of sex drive is associated with social change – you and your partner may be spending more time building careers leaving little time for the pleasures of life, or family pressures from children or elderly parents may preoccupy you. It is also difficult to be interested in sex if you are anxious or depressed.

Vaginal dryness

The other important symptoms of the climacteric occur rather later than the hot flushes and the night sweats. For many women the most important early sign is vaginal dryness, which often occurs alongside painful intercourse, itchiness of the vulva, and an increased propensity for infections. These particular problems do not get better with time, but they can be helped.

Skin

The skin changes. This is because of the loss of collagen from the underside of skin. Collagen is the tough fibre that holds skin together – when cured it becomes leather. But humans do not have that much of it. Despite the fact that there is little of it, however, collagen is important. When it disappears skin wrinkles more, bruises more easily, and in general ages.

Urinary symptoms

In an embryo the tissues that form the lower part of the urinary tract develop from the same cells as the vagina. This means that both structures have similar characteristics, including the fact that oestrogens affect the way they grow. When oestrogens disappear there is weakening of the supporting ligaments, and so urinary problems become important and more common. This can lead to difficulties in controlling urinary flow, or a feeling of urgency, or even episodes of urinary incontinence. These problems can be treated by giving oestrogen or by surgery.

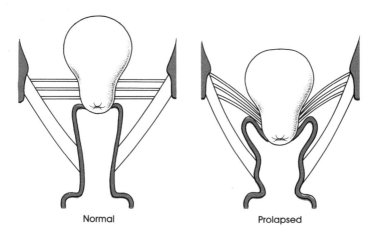

Normal and prolapsed uterus – when oestrogens disappear the supporting ligaments in the vagina become weaker.

How common are these symptoms?

There have been few attempts to study the frequency of these symptoms. They are less common and less severe in fat women than in thin women, but overall about three quarters of all women will get hot flushes. For some women hot flushes will be the only symptoms they get; others will get nearly all of the ones mentioned earlier. A few get symptoms other than hot flushes, but not the flushes themselves.

Research findings

The first study to see how common menopausal symptoms were was carried out in Oxford a few years ago. A researcher studied a group of people who were not actually complaining of menopausal symptoms to their general practitioners. He wanted to see what sorts of things they were really worried about and whether these symptoms were only confined to women approaching the age of 50. Just over 1000 people were contacted to see what health problems they had that they were not necessarily seeing their doctor for. None of those who took part in the study were told that the prime motive for the research was to look at the menopause. The researcher found that both men and women suffered many irritating problems around middle life. Furthermore, many of the individual problems reported were found in up to a third of those contacted. The most impressive findings were the ones that might have been expected; hot flushes and sweats were common in women at the time of the menopause. Interestingly enough, many women also reported that in the years before the menopause they had other problems, such as difficulty in sleeping or loss of confidence. Men did not usually mention any of these problems. Remember, none of these people were told that the researcher was studying the symptoms of the climacteric in women; he made the study look broadly-based.

Some problems disappear after the menopause

The news was not all bad. In women who had passed the menopause many of the health problems they had once had, and which they regarded as trivial, disappeared. These included aching or tingling breasts, irritability, especially when associated with the premenstrual syndrome, and low backache.

The menopause frees many women from some symptoms that come from the ovary and the hormones it produces.

Hormone replacement therapy studies

Questionnaires from researchers are not the only way to study the symptoms of the menopause. If the climacteric is truly a deficiency condition – that is, caused by lack of hormones – then giving the missing hormone to those who have the symptoms of the climacteric should remove those symptoms. Several attempts at this have been carried out and most suggest that replacing oestrogens alleviates the genital symptoms, many of the urinary symptoms, the hot flushes and night sweats, and sometimes the loss of confidence, the loss of memory, and the loss of libido. Giving oestrogens over a longer period prevents the loss of skin texture and bone mineral and protein, and this in turn may remove some of the symptoms such as the difficult to diagnose aches in bones and joints. All of these points are covered in chapter 8.

Preparing for the rest of your life

Listing all of these conditions makes the menopause seem a rather depressing and unpleasant time. You may feel as if your last period marks the first step into senility. But this is not true. Some of the problems and possible long term complications can be helped by treatment. More importantly, the menopause marks the time when careful thought and preparation make the rest of life so much better. Not every woman needs treatment, but every woman needs preparation and the *choice* of receiving or rejecting treatment. Perhaps the most important thing is to have the information that enables you to decide what you want for yourself.

Counselling

Counselling is a much misused word that simply means the giving of information, from someone knowledgeable and understanding, which will help the person being counselled come to the decision that is right for them. To many people who are not trained in counselling, it can seem like a soft option – a few words of sympathy followed by little action. A good counsellor will provide information as well as practical help; this may be simply ways of coping with physical changes, or sorting out career changes, or the possible benefits of hormone replacement therapy. A good counsellor will always collect information about you – he or she cannot counsel in a vacuum and needs to know what is best for you. Counselling is available from menopause clinics, well woman clinics, and family planning clinics, as well as from your family doctor.

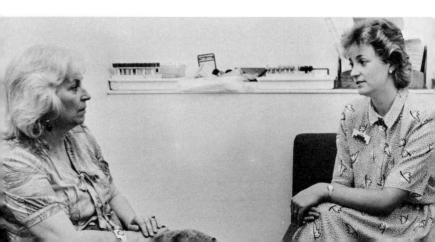

Facing social changes

The years of the climacteric are years of social as well as physical change, and years of reckoning. It is little wonder therefore that you may feel anxious and stressed. It is important to recognise the stressful factors in your life and to develop ways of coping with them so that you don't become unduly anxious, confused, and depressed.

Changing relationships

This is a time of changing family relationships. If you have children, they will be preparing to leave home and at the same time your parents may depend on on you more and more for company or help. And you will have to prepare yourself emotionally for their death. Many people re-assess their marriage now and some partnerships do break up.

Changing self-image

You may have to cope with a changing self-image too. The menopause is not a sign of senility or an indicator that the time has come to relegate yourself (and your sexuality) to the social scrap heap and take up some harmless hobby like tatting or petit point. But it is a time to think very positively about yourself and your life and to look after your own needs. Boost your confidence whenever possible and expand your life through work, voluntary work, or other interests.

A time of reckoning

In these years you realise the extent of the gap between what you wanted to achieve and what is possible now. Don't get down-hearted. Liberate yourself from the past. With all the experience and knowledge you have now, re-assess your aims and goals and look around at new possibilities for the future.

Whatever else you decide, the menopause marks a fundamental change in your life. Things will never be the same again but careful preparation and positive thinking now leads to dividends later.

4 Contraception

Good contraception is perhaps more important at the meno-pause than it is in the rest of a person's life. It needs more thought now than it did earlier because there are some important differences in the suitability of particular methods. Your contraceptive needs change in the years around the menopause, just as they do throughout life and methods suitable for younger women are less suitable now. Gynaeco-logical problems that become apparent for the first time at the menopause may also change contraceptive suitability. All this happens at the same time as the realisation that your fertility (and also menstruation) will be ending soon.

Points to consider

Menstrual irregularity is common as the menopause ap-proaches. For most women this means lighter, less frequent periods but occasionally periods become heavier and longer. This confusing pattern may make you worry about pregnancy and makes methods of family planning that rely on avoiding intercourse at the fertile time of the month less suitable. Nobody likes heavy or long periods, and so anything that makes them worse is unlikely to be welcomed as a contraceptive. Another thing to remember is that some cancers become more common among women in their 50s, and so any contraceptive method that produces irregular bleeding or makes bleeding after intercourse more likely to occur may either worry you unnecessarily or lead you or your doctor to miss an important diagnosis by blaming the irregular bleeding on the contra-ceptive method. There is one other important practical point. During the years before the menopause the falling levels of oestrogen from the ovary often begin to produce some changes in the vagina. There may be a problem with dryness and there is also an increased tendency for infections and an increased likelihood for bleeding after intercourse. All this can make your sex life more uncomfortable and less enjoyable. So what are the best methods of contraception for a woman approaching the menopause?

Contraception is still necessary

The most important point is that contraception is still needed, and will be until a year after the last period. Women are usually less fertile in their 40s, but pregnancy carries more risks at this age than earlier. These health risks are to both the mother and her baby. Also, the irregularity of the periods along with their lightness mean that a pregnancy can be quite advanced before a woman realises she has conceived. This will mean she is then too late for early pregnancy care, for antenatal diagnostic tests such as chorionic villus sampling or amniocentesis, or for abortion, should she want to consider any of these options.

The pill

Three quarters of all women use the oral contraceptive pill at some stage in their lives. Many years ago some research was published that suggested that no one over the age of 35 should take the very high dose oral contraceptive pills that even then were uncommonly used. Unfortunately, this research was misinterpreted and misunderstood and it took many years for the real facts to reach all of the medical profession, let alone the general public. The oral contraceptive pill carries more risks to the health of a woman in her 40s than it does to one in her 20s. But many of these health risks are predictable; they are associated with cigarette smoking, being overweight, having high blood pressure, or having close relatives who have died young from unexpected heart attacks.

Contraceptive pills.

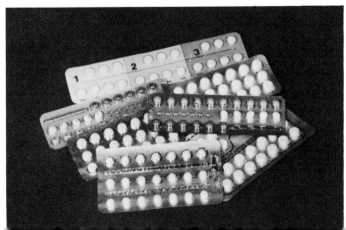

Older women and the pill

For women in the years approaching the menopause the pill is still a good method of contraception. It provides reassurance, it can regulate periods, and the oestrogens in it will offset the falling production of oestrogens from the ovary. Taking oral contraceptives protects against cancer of the ovary and cancer of the endometrium, both of which are more common among women approaching the menopause. Unfortunately, the standard, low dose oral contraceptive pills contain about six times as much hormone as a woman approaching the menopause needs, which is one of the reasons why few women over the age of 45 are suited to the combined oral contraceptive. A few years later, once the menopause has happened, many women start taking oestrogens again but at a much lower dose. This seeming contradiction in advice is discussed again in the chapter on oestrogen hormone replacement treatment.

So for women over the age of 45, or for whom the pill is not suitable, or who do not want to take it, something else is needed. For them, the choice of method is as wide as it was earlier in their life, and for many perhaps wider.

The mini pill

The progestogen only pill, sometimes called the mini pill, does not contain any oestrogen. This makes it suitable for women who are unhappy about taking oestrogens, but this fact also makes it less effective as a contraceptive, especially for younger women. For most women the effect of a progestogen only pill is to make periods lighter and less frequent, which is unlikely to be of much concern to many of those approaching the menopause. For a few women periods become heavier and more frequent, but this is not common, and heavy periods return to normal when the pill is stopped.

Effective for women in their 40s

The arguments about the reduced effectiveness of the progestogen only pill are not relevant to older women and the only studies carried out suggest that it is as effective for women in their 40s as the combined oral contraceptive is for younger women. In other words, you are very unlikely to become pregnant. There is one other advantage to the progestogen only pill; it seems to reduce the frequency of flushes for many, but not all, women.

Intrauterine devices

Although the intrauterine device (IUD) is a widely used contraceptive, it is unsuitable for many young women because it carries an increased risk of failure in this group and is linked with infections in the pelvis, which can lead to infertility. It also causes heavy periods. All of these worries are less of a problem to older women. The IUD is much less likely to be expelled by the uterus of an older woman, especially if she has had children. Pelvic infections such as salpingitis are also less common, and if periods are getting lighter then the effect of the IUD on them is less noticeable.

Contraindications

There are some women, however, for whom the IUD is not suitable. Those with heavy, irregular periods are unlikely to want to use it and so are those with bleeding in between periods. Both of these problems can get worse at this time and since either symptom might suggest the presence of a cancer, unnecessary worry is caused. Both these symptoms need investigation and this usually involves a dilatation and curettage of the uterus (a D&C, or 'scrape'). In this procedure a small sample of the lining of the uterus is scraped away, either under a general anaesthetic in hospital or, more commonly these days, using suction in an outpatients department. Whichever way it is done, any IUD will have to be removed first.

Intrauterine devices (IUDs)

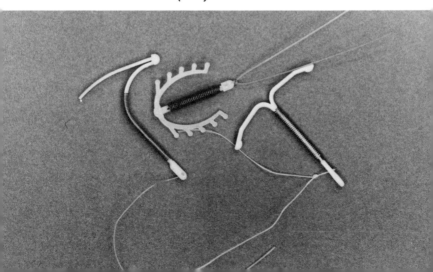

Long-acting hormonal injections

There is one other hormonal contraceptive that you might like to think about – injections of long-acting progestogens. This method has many of the advantages of the progestogen only pill along with the reliability of the IUD but unfortunately it has some disadvantages, which usually make it unsuitable for women in the years of the climacteric.

Controversy

Injections of long-acting progestogens are controversial. There are two forms available in Britain; Depo-Provera and Noristerat. To be effective they need to be injected every two or three months. The idea of injecting contraceptive hormones is not new, and Depo-Provera has been in use for longer than the oral contraceptive pill. Despite this wealth of experience some doctors (although far fewer now than was once the case) are unhappy with these drugs. Their worries relate to two things principally: safety and compulsion.

Areas of concern

Both Depo-Provera and Noristerat are as safe as any other widely used drug. Neither contains oestrogen but despite this both are effective as contraceptives, and are probably as good at stopping pregnancy as the oral contraceptive. Neither has much biochemical effect on the body. The concern that many people have relates to their use in women who may not understand the risks and benefits of them. Young, unsupported mothers still unsure of themselves may be given a long-acting injection without really understanding what it is or why they are being given it. Someone used to dealing with doctors is much less likely to be talked into a drug they may not understand. It is the potential over-use of the drug that arouses much concern.

Drawbacks

Unfortunately, both Depo-Provera and Noristerat have two major drawbacks. Once injected they cannot be removed and both preparations sometimes lead to weight gain and irregular periods. For many women the problems get better (often all they have is light and infrequent periods) but other women get more frequent and heavier periods. Because these drugs often lead to menstrual irregularity, however, they are of less value to most women in the climacteric and are primarily of use to younger women.

Barrier methods

Most women have used barrier contraceptives at some stage of their lives, usually the condom (sheath). Less than 5% of women use the diaphragm or cap regularly but these contraceptives have many advantages for women approaching the menopause. The diaphragm becomes relatively more effective as a contraceptive to women with reduced fertility as they approach the menopause. Another advantage of the diaphragm is that it should be used with a spermicidal cream or jelly. This is considered a disadvantage by many younger women, who see the combination of diaphragms and cream as messy, but spermicides will help older women who may be losing some of their natural vaginal lubrication. Spermicides also help prevent some vaginal infections.

It is important that the cap is fitted properly and spermicidal cream or jelly used.

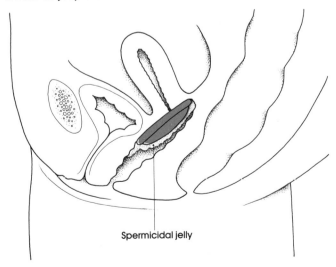

Spermicidal jelly

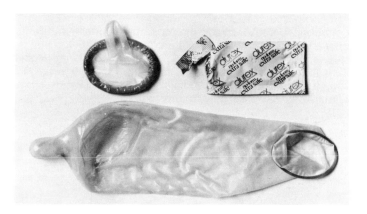

The sheath can be an extremely reliable method of contraception.

Disadvantages

There are some disadvantages. As you approach the menopause problems can develop in the uterus and other genital organs which affect your ability to use a diaphragm. The two most important of these are prolapse and fibroids. Prolapse is a weakening of the supports of the uterus, allowing it to drop downwards through the vagina. Fibroids are growths of muscle that develop in the uterus. They are common, usually harmless, and do little except distort the shape of the uterus. Both can make it difficult to fit and use a diaphragm but neither should prevent its use. Even though a standard diaphragm is unsuitable, an experienced family planning doctor will usually be able to find one that is comfortable and effective.

Sterilisation

Not every woman wants or needs a reversible method of contraception, especially when she is in her late 40s and her family is complete, and so for those the most suitable method of contraception is sterilisation of either the woman or her partner. There was once a suggestion that this was not a good choice for a woman in the last five years of her reproductive life, because the expense and the risks could not be justified in someone who would soon no longer need any method of contraception. Most specialists no longer agree with this; the consequences of an unwanted pregnancy in later life can be devastating and if other forms of contraception are unsuitable, or if the woman wants to be sterilised, then the operation should be offered. On economic grounds sterilisation is cost effective for people of almost any age.

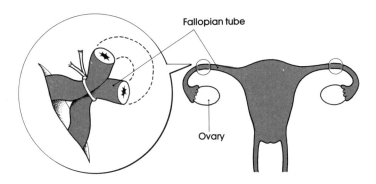

One method of female sterilisation, called tubal ligation, where the fallopian tubes are cut and tied.

Problem of menstrual disturbance

There is one major problem with sterilisation of women. Menstrual disturbances afterwards are common and their cause is unclear. Several studies have suggested that sterilisation has no direct effect on menstruation but there is an indirect effect because women who have been sterilised no longer need a method of contraception. Stopping taking the pill, for example, means that periods become what they would have been if no contraceptive had been used, and this usually means heavier periods than the artificially light ones the pill produces. Another possible explanation for the link between sterilisation and menstrual problems is that periods become much more of a nuisance to a woman once she is no longer able to bear children and so she is much more likely to complain about them.

For whatever reason, many women who have been sterilised report that their periods become heavier and more painful, and blame the operation for this. One in five British women who have been sterilised have a hysterectomy, usually for menstrual problems, in the next 10 years.

Vasectomy

Vasectomy is obviously not a method of contraception for women, but has the reputation of being the most effective contraceptive there is, as well as the only one that has absolutely no effects on women. From the point of view of an individual woman, it is only suitable for those in a stable relationship, but because it is so safe and so effective it is very popular.

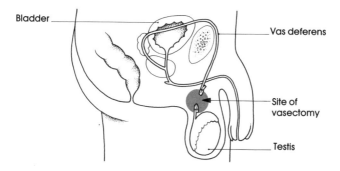

Vasectomy is a minor operation which can be performed under local anaesthetic.

Hysterectomy

There is one other method of contraception sometimes discussed. It combines almost absolute reliability with perfect menstrual control. But hysterectomy (the surgical removal of the uterus) is a major operation, and not usually suggested in Britain simply as a means of stopping the risk of pregnancy.

The abdominal approach

Hysterectomy is carried out using one of two routes. The traditional method used in Britain for many years was for the surgeon to make a cut in the front of the abdomen, and through this remove the uterus, leaving behind the ovaries. There is usually a stay in hospital of about a week, with up to two months recuperation afterwards.

37

Vaginal approach

More gynaecologists are now turning to an alternative method of performing the operation. In this approach, the operation is carried out through the vagina, and again the uterus is removed, while the ovaries are usually left behind. This technique has several advantages over the older one. There is no scar on the front of the abdomen. There is less disturbance to the rest of the body, and so there is less pain after the operation, and women are usually able to go home from hospital sooner. The other important point is that operating using this approach allows the treatment of prolapse, because the supports of the vagina and bladder can be tightened if this is necessary.

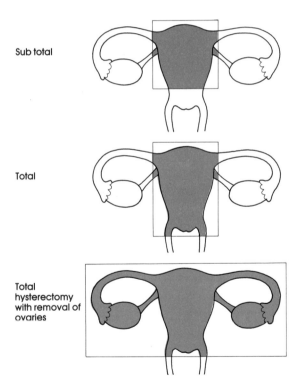

Sub total

Total

Total
hysterectomy
with removal of
ovaries

The different types of hysterectomy.

Effective but drastic

Hysterectomy is an effective, but perhaps drastic, method of contraception. It is said to prevent the subsequent development of cancer of the uterus as well as cancer of the ovaries (even if the ovaries have been left behind; the reason for this protection is uncertain). It certainly makes oestrogen hormone replacement treatment easier to give, because there is no longer any concern about the effect of hormones on the endometrium, and it always controls menstrual problems. Few doctors, however, would recommend a hysterectomy simply for these reasons.

Give contraception serious thought

Whatever you think about contraception, think about it again now. Talk it over with your GP, and if you want a second opinion, talk it over with someone in a family planning clinic. Don't rush your decision but do make one – the consequences of an unwanted pregnancy are even more serious now than they once were.

Unprotected intercourse

If you do have unprotected intercourse go and see your doctor straight away. He or she may prescribe the 'morning after pill' – a combined oestrogen/progestogen pill. Alternatively they may insert an IUD into your uterus. This is very effective if carried out up to five days after unprotected intercourse.

Discuss the following types of contraception with your GP to decide which is best for you or your partner:

The pill	**Barrier Methods**
	Cap
Intrauterine devices	**Sheath**
Hormonal injections	**Vasectomy**
Sterilisation	**Hysterectomy**

5 Osteoporosis

Much of what has been written and said in the past about the menopause has been controversial. There is one fact, however, about which there is almost no argument – the menopause marks that time in a woman's life when not only the amount of material in each bone she has begins to decline, but the bone that is left weakens too. This process is called osteoporosis. Osteoporosis means that bones become more likely to break if there are sudden stresses or deform if stresses are slight and continuous. Osteoporosis does not occur in every woman but perhaps one in four who live long enough will be affected by it. The stresses that damage bones need not be great – for some women turning over in bed is enough to break their hip bones – and the breaks need not be as obvious as the word implies. Small crush fractures of the vertebrae may be unnoticed except on x-rays; the gradual squashing of vertebrae may do little more than make the woman shorter than she once was, or lead to the stooped back and difficulty in looking straight ahead that caricaturises old age and was once termed the 'Dowager's hump'.

A subject of argument

The arguments about preventing osteoporosis begin after that short statement of fact. In every branch of medicine, professionals, the public, and those who have to pay the bills, agree that prevention is always better than attempting a cure. The problem is that prevention of osteoporosis is not easy, but since there is not really a cure either the controversy about prevention is going to continue for a long time. This chapter is about current thinking on osteoporosis and its prevention, but in the end the best way for a woman to prevent osteoporosis is to take charge of her own body.

How big is the problem?

Every year in the United States of America one million bones are broken in women who have gone through the menopause. Half of these broken bones are vertebrae, one fifth wrist and lower arm bones, and one third of them hip bones. The total cost of treating these women is about $6 billion annually. The figures in the United Kingdom are similar – the NHS spends at least £2 million every week on fractured hips alone. In fact, the third commonest reason for admission to a non-psychiatric hospital in Britain is a fractured hip.

Consequences to the individual

These figures are bad but even worse are the consequences for the women involved. Hip fractures are the most serious, and as a result of these between 10 and 15% of women will die, either immediately or within a few months of being admitted to hospital. There are also long term disabilities, with as many as half of the women being affected badly, sometimes so badly that they are unable to live independently, and either have to go and live with relatives or move into residential homes. Whatever happens, the fracture will permanently affect the quality of their lives.

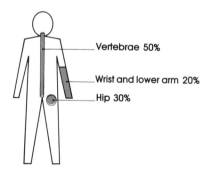

Vertebrae 50%

Wrist and lower arm 20%

Hip 30%

Bones particularly at risk from osteoporosis.

Every day 14 women in Britain die as a result of a hip fracture.

Wrist fractures are distressing too

The problem is not only fractures of the hip. Even something that would be regarded by doctors and a woman's friends and relatives as trivial, such as a broken wrist, has long term consequences. After such an injury and the pain and sometimes the indignity of having to wait in a strange hospital casualty department for the bones to be set, many people become scared of leaving the house (especially in winter when the pavements are slippery) in case something similar happens again. All fractures heal less well in older people, and so women who have broken their wrists may be troubled by pain and be unable to make careful wrist movements for far longer than someone younger. This might not sound like much of a problem but imagine trying to cook, dress, drive, or make a pot of tea with only one usable wrist.

Why do bones break?

Bones are like everything else – they break when they are overstressed. But bones in older people, and especially older women, resist stress less well and break more easily. There are many reasons for this relative weakness but also important as a cause of fracture and injury is the way that age imposes additional stresses.

Stresses of age

Older people tend to move less briskly than younger people and they sometimes have handicaps such as poor eyesight or joint stiffness that make them less able to move freely. Their reflexes are slower than those of young people. This explains why even though they move around less they are more likely to fall over, and why one fifth of the broken bones in women over the age of 50 are in the wrist: they fall, and put their hands out to save themselves, which was safe when they were younger, but now their hands and wrists take the brunt of the damage.

Exercise is important

Every part of the body is being renewed all the time. Just as old blood cells are broken down and their proteins and other chemicals reused by the body, so bone is being continually remodelled. This happens in cycles in small areas where one tiny patch is broken down, and then over the next few months rebuilt, while another focus elsewhere is broken down and the proteins and minerals recirculated. From the first moment of breakdown to the final remineralisation takes about two years. This leads to the difficulty in treating and studying the problem; any research will take many years to see if a new treatment is working. In women who have not reached their 40s the net effect is for the amount of bone (the 'bone mass') to increase gradually, with the increase greatest in the areas where the stresses are greatest. In other words, if bones are being used, they grow stronger, especially at the points where they face stresses and so need to be strongest. If they are not being stressed they weaken gradually.

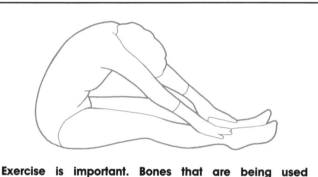

Exercise is important. Bones that are being used grow stronger, if bones are not being stressed they weaken gradually.

The process of bone loss

At some stage in their 40s, bone renewal changes for both men and women, but the effect is much more pronounced in women. Gradually the rate of bone loss becomes the same as that of bone building, and eventually established bone disappears faster than new bone is formed. Since the rate at which bone is lost is relatively constant, women who start this process with dense strong bones will still have relatively more bone after 10 years than someone who enters the years after the menopause with less bone. Between the age of 40 and death, men lose 20% of the protein and mineral material that make up their bones, while women lose 35%. Not all of this difference is because of the hormonal changes that accompany the menopause, because on average women live longer than men, and so have more time to lose bone material. At similar ages women have less material in their bones than men do.

How can osteoporosis be prevented?

All of this information leads to three ideas for preventing osteoporosis.

- The most obvious is that if bones can be strengthened before the rate of bone loss overtakes that of new bone formation, then because the person is starting from a higher level it will mean their bones are always somewhat stronger than they would be if they had weaker bones at the start of the process.
- A second idea is that if the building materials for bones can always be present in excess then even if bone loss is continuing perhaps bone rebuilding will not be hampered. The analogy here is with a factory; if the raw materials are kept in constant high supply then production will never fail. Just as the story does not work for all factories so it doesn't seem to work for all people, except perhaps those with poor nutrition who show some improvement in bone formation when their diet gets better.
- And finally, if the reason women lose bone at a faster rate than men is the failing ovary, then reversing or side-stepping that failure will make sure that bone growth continues at the rate it did before the menopause.

Who is most likely to be affected by osteoporosis?

Osteoporosis is more likely to occur in some women than others, although the most important single indicator is age, and especially age since the menopause. There are some other factors that predict an increased risk for osteoporosis but most of them are relatively unimportant.

Risk factors for osteoporosis

- Women who are white or of Indian/Pakistani origin;
- Women who have mothers or sisters who had severe and early osteoporosis;
- Women who have always had a poor intake of calcium (for example, Vegans);
- Women who are underweight or suffer from anorexia nervosa;
- Women who had an early menopause, or removal of both ovaries when young (unless they took additional or replacement oestrogens);
- Women who have a diet high in phosphate;
- Women who have, or have had, a sedentary life-style;
- Women who have never had children;
- Women who drink a lot of alcohol;
- Women who smoke cigarettes;
- Women who have a diet high in protein;
- Women who drink a lot of caffeine;
- Women who have a high salt intake.

Interrelated risk factors

Some of these factors are interrelated. As an example, dietary calcium and phosphate are linked, because a diet rich in phosphate will lead to calcium phosphate being formed in the intestine, which the body is unable to absorb, making the effect on the body similar to a diet deficient in calcium. Similarly, cigarette smoking makes the ovaries work less efficiently, and so the net effect is to make the menopause begin earlier, and the ovaries produce fewer hormones than normal in the years before the menopause. Cigarette smoking also acts directly on the cells that produce new bone.

Some question marks

Other factors are not understood. Chinese women appear to develop osteoporosis less frequently than women from other parts of Asia. This might be related to a genetic difference, or it might be something of dietary origin. Black women also seem to be relatively immune to osteoporosis, and this may be because in general they do much more hard physical work than white women, or it may be because of a genetic difference in bone mass at maturity between black and other women. It has been pointed out that although black athletes dominate much of the track and field events all over the globe there are few world-class black swimmers, and that this may be because a higher bone-mass in black athletes gives them athletic strength and endurance, but makes swimming more difficult because they are less buoyant in water.

Can osteoporosis be prevented?

Osteoporosis probably cannot be prevented in everybody, but its effects can be minimised, reducing the chances of an individual woman being badly affected. Many of these preventative measures are simple, and are easy for you to carry out by yourself. Unfortunately, these measures alone will not have a major effect, and the most efficient and effective preventative measure involves the use of hormone treatment. The use of oestrogen hormone replacement to prevent long term problems is still argued about. Almost all specialists in the field accept that it is effective, and probably better than anything else likely to be developed over the next two decades. But its main effects are going to be felt many years after the menopause, and some women are concerned that they might have to take hormones for 20 years to get the full benefit of them. These arguments are weighed up in the chapter on hormone treatment after the menopause. Here we will discuss simpler techniques. Remember, the most important way these methods work is to improve the quality of bone and the amount of it; ideally they should be used for 10 or 20 years *before* the menopause.

Exercise

Everybody accepts that exercise is good for you, and so lots of exercise must be even better. Unfortunately, that is not quite true. Most types of exercise lead to an increase in the amount of bone formed, and in general terms, women who are athletic or who do hard physical work tend to have stronger bones than those who demand less of their bodies. There is an important exception. Women who are excessively athletic, such as female athletes or ballet dancers, sometimes develop osteoporosis and break bones despite their exercise. This apparent contradiction happens because a combination of the strict diets that athletes and ballet dancers need, along with their exercise, leads to a condition somewhat similar to anorexia nervosa. The important feature of this condition is that their ovaries tend not to function normally, and so the women do not ovulate, which means little oestrogen hormone production, and eventually osteoporosis similar to that of women some years after the menopause. All this means that for most women some exercise will strengthen bones, but too much, along with a lack of oestrogen, may actually damage them.

> **Too little exercise will not weaken bones to the point where osteoporosis sets in, but it will make osteoporosis more likely to develop earlier in the years after the menopause.**

Type of exercise is important

One interesting development of the past years has been the realisation that one group of people, few of them women, are at great risk from what appears to their bones as lack of exercise. People flying in space often have to work very hard, but the absence of gravity means that despite the exercise they do, their bones develop severe osteoporosis. The lesson for earth women is that the most efficient exercises to help prevent osteoporosis are those which act against gravity. Walking and running are better for you than swimming. Exercise in people who already have osteoporosis can be dangerous while the bones are still being strengthened; repetitive stress, for example something like jogging, can lead to bones being crushed or fractured. The corollary is that people with osteoporosis should be kept active; if they break a bone it should be treated quickly and in such a way as to make sure they keep mobile. Three months in hospital with a broken leg will be unpleasant for a young man who has had a car accident; it could be fatal for a 65 year old woman who has had a fall at home.

It doesn't have to be unpleasant

Exercise does not have to be unpleasant physical jerks at a keep fit class or expensive sessions at a gymnasium. Women who own large dogs and take them for regular walks, strengthen their own skeletons. So do women who live in houses with at least one flight of stairs, because the regular going up and down is again excellent, although repetitive, exercise.

There is one other way that exercise is important. Any exercise that keeps people active, and in control of their lives, and physically coordinated, may make falls less likely to occur, as well as strengthening the underlying bone.

One disadvantage

Exercise to prevent osteoporosis does present one problem – you need a lot of it for a long period of time. If you want to take your exercise as walking, for instance, you will need to walk at least an additional 30 miles a week to have a good effect on your bones. If you have a full time job, or even if you don't, that is a lot of extra time devoted to exercise. It is the search for an easier solution that has made so many people concentrate on diet and drugs.

Diet

Before the menopause women take in more calcium in their diet than they pass out in their urine and stools. After the menopause this reverses. The rate at which calcium is absorbed from the diet depends partly on the form it is in (some forms of calcium cannot be absorbed), the amount of it present, the presence of other things in the diet that prevent the calcium being absorbed, the health of the stomach and intestine (40% of women over the age of 50 have little acid in their stomachs between meals, and so if they take calcium tablets then the additional calcium will be ineffective, because acid is needed for the calcium to be absorbed) and the presence of vitamin D. Vitamin D comes partly from the diet, and partly from the conversion of other chemicals to Vitamin D in the skin under the influence of sunlight.

Overweight is a two-edged sword

Overeating to the point of being overweight is a two-edged sword. In general, fat women have more oestrogens and so are less prone to osteoporosis. They carry more weight onto their skeletons, which helps them too: But they also tend to move less, which is not good for the bones, and they are more prone to heart disease. So, don't get anorexia, but don't get overweight either!

The truth about calcium

All of these factors combine to make it difficult to be sure about the usefulnes of changing or improving the amount of calcium in the diet to prevent osteoporosis. The scientific evidence is confused, and many (but certainly not all) studies have shown no practical benefits from taking additional calcium. If it does work, then it works best in younger women. At the same time no treatment or prevention of osteoporosis is going to work if your diet is deficient in calcium. So perhaps the most sensible thing to say is that *men and women in their 50s and beyond should eat more dairy products, such as yoghurt or cheese, and if they are unhappy about this take additional calcium tablets, but take them with meals* because then the calcium is more likely to be absorbed. None of this will be harmful, but it is much more beneficial to ensure that your diet is good in the decades before the menopause.

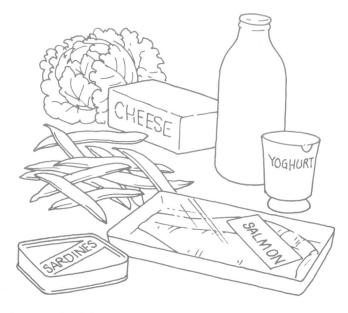

Sources of calcium

Other factors that help or hinder

Both smoking cigarettes and drinking alcohol damage bone production. Cigarettes do this by reducing the production of oestrogens from the ovary and also by acting directly on the cells in bones that actually produce new bone. Alcohol probably acts directly on the bone production cells, but it also affects the liver which helps control blood hormone levels.

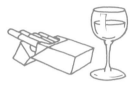

Alcohol and cigarettes damage bone production.

Fluoride

Fluoride strengthens bone, and so some women take supplements of sodium fluoride. Excessive amounts of fluoride make bone thicker but not stronger, but in small amounts the development of osteoporosis is halted. Cities that put fluoride in their water supply have fewer women who develop osteoporosis.

Drugs that may not help

Some years ago, hot flushes and other aches and pains of ageing were treated with sedatives and tranquilisers. This practice has generally been abandoned, but anybody who receives drugs of this type for any other reason is much more likely to fall, as well as being less likely to get additional exercise.

Look after your feet

One other simple factor that is often forgotten is chiropody and footwear. Women with painful feet are less likely to walk around, and so more likely to develop osteoporosis, and when they do walk they are more likely to hobble and fall, and so break bones. Similarly, poorly fitting shoes, or shoes with poor grips, are more likely to make women not want to go for walks, or slip when they do.

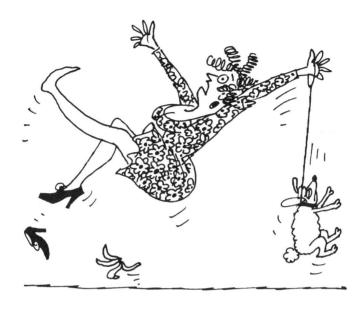

Drugs

Drugs may act by increasing the formation of new bone or preventing the dissolution of existing bone. Many drugs and combinations of drugs have been tried, but the only ones that seem to be effective are oestrogen hormone replacement, calcium, and calcitonin. Calcium tablets have been mentioned before, and oestrogens will be discussed in a later chapter of this book.

Calcitonin

Calcitonin is a normal body hormone produced by the parathyroid glands. It acts on the cells that normally absorb bone, and prevents them from working. This means that its usefulness in treating established osteoporosis is minimal, but it may have a role in preventing it. It may be useful with something else that acts to build up bone strength. Calcitonin is a protein, and so cannot be given by mouth, which also limits its effectiveness.

Practical ways to help

Osteoporosis can be made less of a nightmare. But preparation for it and its prevention begins almost half a century before it is likely to exist. So however old you are, there is no time to lose.

- Make sure that children, particularly girls, have a good diet with lots of calcium, and lots of exercise, so that they go into adulthood with a good skeleton.
- Adults, especially those over 50, should keep active. Care in their own homes is much more likely to keep people active than care in a residential home. If bones break, try to get them fixed surgically and soon.
- Keep your diet rich in calcium.
- Keep your weight normal.
- Stop smoking, and keep alcohol consumption under control.
- Keep some exposure to sunshine.
- Read the chapter on oestrogen hormone replacement therapy, and make up your own mind on the risks and benefits.

6 Heart and blood vessel disease

Diseases of the heart and blood vessels lead to problems such as strokes and heart attacks, and they are common and important. But the problem is not simply one of death. (Most people would agree that a sudden heart attack is perhaps one of the more pleasant ways to die – if any way of dying can ever be said to be pleasant.) Heart disease also causes a lot of disability and pain, and not only to the patient. A family can be devastated if a parent has a stroke or becomes disabled by severe and continual pain from heart or blood vessel disease. Treatment of most forms of heart disease is not very successful, and prevention of even a small proportion of heart attacks would improve the state of the nation's health more than almost anything else. Unfortunately, preventing heart disease is much more boring than treating it, and so has a low priority in most health programmes. If you want to prevent heart disease, you will have to take charge of your own body.

Diseases of the heart and blood vessels are the most important cause of death among British people.

Who gets heart disease?

Although heart disease is important, it is often not unexpected. Some women are more likely to develop heart disease than others and if you are one of them, then, strangely enough, you are lucky – lucky because if you know you are at a special risk of a heart attack or a stroke you can do something about it.

Risk factors

Women at particular risk are:

- Those who smoke;
- Those whose partners smoke;
- Those who are overweight;
- Those who have high blood pressure;
- Those who take little exercise;
- Those who have had close family relatives die young of heart disease;
- Those who went through the menopause relatively early.

Since you cannot control the last two points, if they apply to you it means you should take additional care of your health. Drinking alcohol makes strokes more likely to occur but does not seem to change the incidence of heart attacks, although by increasing weight it indirectly makes them more likely to happen.

The epidemiology of heart disease

Heart disease is so important that much medical and scientific effort has been put into studying its epidemiology. In epidemiology, medical scientists use the techniques once used to study epidemics of infectious disease to describe the collection and analysis of as much information as possible about any disease. They hope that by using this information they can understand how a particular disease starts and then develop ways of treating or preventing it.

Study results

When these techniques were applied to heart disease, several interesting points were found. The first is that although heart disease is uncommon among women before the menopause, things begin to change after it. Women do not get severe heart disease as commonly as men, however, until they both reach the age of 75. Usually, the only women who develop serious heart or blood vessel disease before the menopause are those who have some other health problem such as diabetes, or women who smoke. Even for these women though, heart disease seems milder than in those men who have the same risk factors. The risk of heart disease in women is not entirely related to age. Most diseases become more common as people age but heart disease is more prevalent among women who have stopped menstruating than among women of the same age who are still having periods.

Why are postmenopausal women susceptible?

So what are the special reasons for this sudden change in susceptibility to heart disease? There are two obvious changes in women at the menopause – their periods stop and oestrogen hormone production declines.

Menstruation affects blood clotting

Women are always a little more anaemic than men, and it was once believed that menstruation caused this. Since all the blood a woman loses in a year through menstruation would fit into a pint milk bottle, however, and since blood donors give twice that amount a year without any effect on their health this belief is probably incorrect. But the fact remains that women are more anaemic than men and, for whatever reason, people who are slightly anaemic seem less likely to develop blood clots. 'Thinner' blood seems to go round the body faster than does the blood of someone who is not anaemic. Both of these points might make heart attacks and strokes less likely to occur. Menstruation is associated with some changes in the way blood clots and it is just possible that this helps in the prevention of heart attacks.

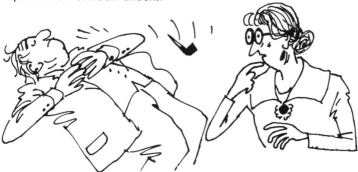

Hormonal changes

Much more important are the hormone changes that occur with the menopause. All hormones from the ovary affect the rest of the body and one of their important effects is on the way the body breaks down and uses fat – both directly and through the effects of oestrogen on the production of fat carrier proteins (molecules that transport fat from one part of the body to another). Fat is important both as part of the diet where it provides energy but also as a building block for many structures in the body, ranging from hormones to cell membranes. Not all the fat in the body comes from the food we eat; some is made from other constituents of the diet. Too little fat in the blood stream is as harmful as too much. Part of the harm that diabetes does comes from the abnormalities it produces in the way the body handles fats.

Lipoproteins

One of the most important fats is cholesterol. Cholesterol is needed as the basis for many hormones but the cells of the body that need it most are unable to make it from the basic building chemicals in the diet. Like all fats, cholesterol does not dissolve in water, and so it is carried in the blood stream (which is mostly water) by the special carrier proteins. There is an entire family of these proteins, called lipoproteins, and medical scientists tell them apart by the way they settle in centrifuge tubes – the heaviest, which sink to the bottom fastest, are the high density lipoproteins (HDL); the next are the low density lipoproteins (LDL); and then come the very low density lipoproteins (VLDL).

Lipoproteins and cholesterol levels

Most of the body's cholesterol is carried by the HDL which not only carry the cholesterol but will also scavenge and bind to free cholesterol. Free cholesterol, which is simply cholesterol not bound to carrier proteins, when present in excess will settle in blood vessel walls, and these collections are the start of the furring or thickening of blood vessels called 'atherosclerosis'. If there are a lot of HDL they will mop up any excess cholesterol, prevent it from damaging the lining of the blood vessels, and carry it to the liver where it is broken down into the bile acids that assist digestion. Several good epidemiological studies have shown that people with high levels of HDL have less heart disease than those with normal or low levels of HDL, perhaps because they have less free cholesterol damaging their blood vessels.

Oestrogen and lipoproteins

Production of all lipoproteins is partly controlled by the oestrogens in the blood, and the decline in hormone production after the menopause may be responsible for the changes in lipoprotein levels and the fact that within a few years of the menopause heart disease becomes much more common in women. It takes over 20 years for the rates of heart disease to become the same in both sexes, but this would fit in with the slow development of atherosclerosis after the change in lipoprotein levels.

Oestrogens and heart disease

The first attempts to stop heart disease by giving oestrogens were depressing. Men who had had at least one heart attack were given additional oestrogens, usually in the form of tablets of the powerful synthetic hormone diethyl-stilboestrol. Many suffered unpleasant side effects and yet despite this the drug did not seem to prevent disease; in fact, the men who took the tablets had more heart attacks and died sooner than men who did not receive the drugs.

How strokes happen.

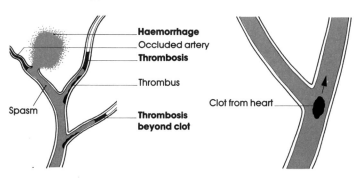

Haemorrhage
Occluded artery
Thrombosis
Thrombus
Spasm
Thrombosis beyond clot
Clot from heart

Why did this happen?

There are lots of possible reasons for this disappointing result but perhaps the most important was that giving men powerful, synthetic, female hormones in high doses is not sensible; it is certainly not the same as trying to replicate smaller changes occurring in women after the menopause. Synthetic oestrogens have side effects. They raise blood pressure, which damages the heart and blood vessels and they make blood more likely to clot inside blood vessels, which leads to heart attacks or strokes if that clot reaches the heart or brain. Not only is the type of oestrogen important, however, so is the way it is given. This is an important aspect that will be covered in the chapter on oestrogen hormone replacement.

More research

While all this was being puzzled over, another piece of research that seemed to contradict earlier studies was published. It pointed out that men who had high blood levels of oestrogen had more heart disease than men with low levels. This seemed to suggest that oestrogens caused heart disease. Apart from the obvious errors of trying to study heart disease in women by looking at hormone levels in men, there is one other flaw in this study. As oestrogen is formed in fat cells men with high blood levels of oestrogen tended to be fat. Fatness is itself an important cause of heart disease, and so there was a confounding factor accounting for much of the difference. Men who have high blood oestrogen levels because of an extra chromosome do not get more heart disease than other men. And, even more importantly, men who go on a strict, fat free diet lose weight, achieve lower blood cholesterol levels, and get lower blood levels of oestrogen as well.

Oestrogens and women

So, are oestrogens good for women? Until recently, the story seemed confusing. When women's oestrogen production went down their lipoprotein levels changed, and later they got heart disease as commonly as men. When men were given oestrogens, they got heart disease. So what happened when women were given oestrogens?

Again, until recently, the story was confused. Young women who smoked and were given high doses of synthetic oestrogens, such as were present in the early versions of the oral contraceptive pill, certainly developed heart disease and had strokes. This picture coloured research for many years. There are, however, some special points to make. In young women, oestrogens lead to clots in the blood vessels, which may cause strokes. They also lead to high blood pressure which can result in heart disease. High doses of synthetic hormones, along with cigarette smoking, therefore seem to be harmful to this group.

But what about those older women who no longer have their own supply of oestrogens? And those who are taking low doses of natural oestrogens without added hormones like progestogens that might themselves cause heart disease? There have been more arguments about the link between the menopause and heart disease and the use of oestrogens in menopausal women and heart disease than about almost any other aspect of the menopause. Some of the facts are simple. Giving oestrogens improves the pattern of lipoproteins in the blood. Will that improve the health of women? For years researchers have been saying that it probably will, but that more research is needed.

Any answers?

The answer seems to be emerging now. The earlier concerns about oestrogens and men, and oestrogens in high doses and young smoking women, do not seem to be relevant for much lower doses of oestrogens given to women who have passed the menopause. Several large studies, such as one looking at the health of over 100 000 American nurses, seem to suggest that for women who do not smoke and who take low dose oestrogens, there is a great deal of benefit. Heart attacks and strokes are much less common. The story will not end here, however. There is already one interesting point for future analysis – does the progestogen component of hormone replacement therapy lead to an increased risk of heart disease? (A progestogen is a synthetic drug that mimics the hormone progesterone and is often given with oestrogens.) That question may well be answered in a future edition of this book!

Reducing the risk of heart attack

The first obvious step you should take is to look for risk factors and then avoid those that can be avoided. Anyone who has ever tried to lose weight knows how difficult that is. Exercise can be a problem too – we don't all have the time for as much as we want and need. The most dangerous thing of all, however, is to smoke or live with someone who does. There is no such thing as a safe cigarette or even a safe number to smoke every day. Stop for your heart's sake or your partner's sake. After you have tried to eliminate these risk factors, consider the use of oestrogens. But don't be tempted to look for easy solutions – the simple pill to take, rather than the difficult decisions about diet, exercise and smoking.

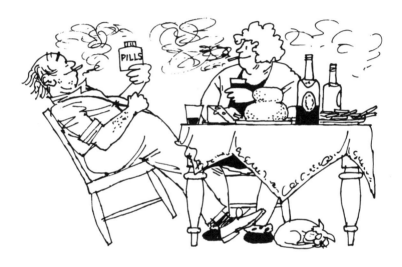

7 Treatment options

The last few chapters may seem pretty depressing to you. The menopause seems to mark the end of your immunity to heart disease, the beginning of osteoporosis, and the end of your sexuality. Can you prevent these changes? Does the menopause need 'treatment'? Is it a 'disease' that should make you go straight to your doctor and ask for medicine?

A complex problem

There is no easy answer to that question. The rest of this book will try and provide answers and if you decide you do want some form of medical treatment, it will tell you about the sorts of treatment you can get, and how to go about getting them.

The first and most important point to make is that although changes are going to happen in your body, you can prepare for them and make them less troublesome. You can prepare for them by changing your diet and by increasing the amount of exercise you take. But if you want to replace the oestrogens that you are no longer producing, the only way is by taking them as medicines. It was once argued that this is unnatural, but then so is living in cities. If the menopause is regarded as a deficiency condition, then treatment is as sensible as treating thyroid insufficiency. You might not want to take hormone treatment, however, so what other options are there?

Treatments other than hormone replacement

When the level of oestrogen in the blood falls, symptoms develop. These include hot flushes, night sweats, vaginal dryness, and ultimately loss of bone mineral. There is not really any guaranteed, effective treatment for night sweats and hot flushes other than oestrogen replacement. But if you cannot or do not want to take oestrogens, and do not want to endure the symptoms, the options available include evening primrose oil, clonidine, and tranquilisers or sedatives.

Progestogens

Some women have tried progestogens, drugs that will break down in the body to have an effect similar to the hormone progesterone. Progestogens do not have many of the side effects of oestrogen, but then neither do they have many of the benefits. There is not really much place for them on their own in the treatment of the climacteric. Some women find that progestogens help reduce the frequency of hot flushes.

Tranquilisers

Tranquilisers and sedatives do not really have a place at all in treating the symptoms of the climacteric and will almost certainly do more harm than good. Their use harks back to a time when keeping people quiet was considered the best way of dealing with their problems.

Evening primrose oil

Evening primrose oil is rich in unsaturated fatty acids, mainly linoleic and linolenic acids. It has been suggested as a panacea for many ills from skin disease to arthritis, and has also been suggested as a treatment for the premenstrual syndrome and some of the symptoms of the menopause. It is of unproved benefit, but probably safe.

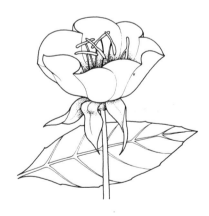

The evening primrose.

Clonidine

Clonidine (Dixarit) is a drug sometimes used to treat high blood pressure. It has other effects on the body, however, one of which is to act on blood vessels to prevent flushes. It works, and works well, but does not treat the other symptoms of the climacteric. It has no effect on the hormonal deficiency.

Diet and exercise

Prevention of osteoporosis has already been covered. The important points to make again are that exercise in the years before the menopause leads to an increase not only in the strength of bones, but also in the amount of bone the body has. Inevitably, some bone is lost over the next few decades, but women who start the process of losing bone with stronger bones containing more protein and mineral will not lose as much, or lose it as fast, as those who start with weaker bones. A good diet, with additional calcium and vitamin D, helps to increase the amount of calcium in the skeleton, but diet alone will never increase the strength of the skeleton.

Oestrogen hormone replacement therapy

So this brings us back to the question of hormones. Should you take them? Oestrogens will usually prevent vaginal dryness, hot flushes and night sweats, much of the loss of bone mineral from the skeleton, the loss of collagen from the skin, and they may help to prevent depression. But taking oestrogens will also mean that your periods will return, that you may also suffer from premenstrual syndrome, and the risk of developing cancer of the endometrium and breast is greater. So should you take hormone replacement? The next chapter tries to provide you with some of the answers.

8 Hormone replacement therapy

Why should you take hormone replacement therapy?

For some questions, it is not possible to give the same answer to everyone and this is one such question. There are good reasons for every woman to consider taking hormone replacement treatment, and there are good reasons why no one should take it. But the final decision must come down to you – it's your body and your choice. This chapter is about taking hormones, principally oestrogens, after you have passed the menopause. It discusses the types of hormones you may take, the good points and the bad points.

Why a menopause anyway?

Before trying to answer the question about why women might want to take hormones there is an anthropological or philosophical point to consider. There are still no really good explanations for the menopause. Why should the ovary fail to continue producing hormones for as long as a woman lives? In most of the animal kingdom, a being that loses the ability to reproduce dies. Humans are different, however, they have life after reproduction. They share this ability with few other animals, as none of the other primates have anything like the menopause. But the animals regarded by some as our next closest relatives, the toothed whales (animals such as the dolphin), do.

A social reason

There is probably a social reason for the menopause. It almost certainly exists to allow women who have knowledge and experience to pass that on to their children and their children's children. If experienced or knowledgeable women continued to be fertile they would continue to have children themselves, and devote themselves to their own families. Perhaps the greatest advantage for the survival of the species, or the genes of the species, is for older women to help with the care and education of younger members of society, rather than continuing to produce their own. This is one explanation for the menopause. It implies that the menopause follows social development, and as an explanation it is as good as any other.

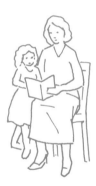

A hormone and egg situation!

If this explanation is correct, it begins to explain the reasons for the menopause and why it is associated with the failure of the ovaries to produce hormones, which in turn leads to unpleasant symptoms and a worsening of the quality of life for many women after the age of 50. In women, as in most of the animal kingdom, the ovaries have evolved to produce both hormones and eggs, and the two functions are not really separable. Unfortunately, when the ability to produce eggs stops, hormones and the control they provide also stop.

Changing the question

This means that the original question needs to be changed. Women have to decide for themselves, 'Should I interfere with something predestined and give myself the hormones my body lacks?' It is a personal, not a medical, question.

Analogous situations

There is an analogy with two other problems the body faces, although the analogy is not really a fair one. In both diabetes mellitus and myxoedema the body fails to produce enough hormones. In diabetes, the pancreas fails to produce the hormone insulin and in myxoedema the thyroid gland does not produce the hormones it should. When people get either of these diseases they are treated with the missing hormones and this has led some enthusiasts to suggest that the same should be true of ovarian failure. But neither myxoedema nor diabetes occur in everyone, or even half the population, while every woman who lives long enough goes through the menopause. Untreated diabetes is fatal and thyroid deficiency can lead to death. The menopause does not kill, although it may hasten death by increasing the rates at which women get heart and blood vessel disease. Despite this postmenopausal increase in death rates, however, women still live longer than men, on average.

Elixir of life?

Almost since history began people have been trying to prevent ageing. Mediaeval alchemists spent much of their lives searching for the elixir of life. Myths surround the quest for the eternal life. The goddess Aurora gave her mortal lover Tithonus eternal life, but forgot to ask for eternal youth for him; he aged but could not die.

Monkey glands

The use of hormones to reverse or prevent some of the consequences of ageing has been suggested for centuries. In the United States in the last century men would eat bulls' testes to improve their potency and try to prevent old age developing. These testes contained some male sex hormones but not in a form that could be absorbed easily, and not really enough anyway to have much of an effect. The sex hormones a bull produces are essentially the same as those produced by male humans.

Earlier this century there was a similar vogue for injections and transplants of extracts of monkey glands (again, the testes of monkeys). They were prescribed for both men and women and were alleged to have similar beneficial effects. Giving them by injection was more effective than swallowing them but even then they were not particularly effective and enthusiasm waned.

Advances in endocrinology

None of these treatments was studied scientifically, and eventually all fell into disrepute. Hormone treatment was used intermittently until the advances in endocrinology (the study of hormones) that came about in the early part of this century gave medical scientists the ability to purify hormones, initially from animals. This meant that for the first time measured doses of hormones could be given and their effects noted. This demonstrated that women who had no hormones showed a dramatic response when given them. Another interesting side to this is that since most of the early work on the use of hormones to treat the menopause was carried out using hormones from animals, these are still the most studied and most widely used hormones.

Hormone treatments

Three hormones used in the treatment of symptoms of the climacteric are:

● Oestrogens
● Progestogens
● Testosterone.

Oestrogens are the principal hormones used in menopausal hormone replacement treatment but given on their own they can be dangerous. Oestrogens lead to overgrowth of the endometrium and progesterone is needed to prevent this. This is discussed later, but because progesterone is poorly absorbed by the body and rapidly broken down when it is absorbed, it is rarely used in treatment – drugs called progestogens that have a similar effect in the body are given instead. Although testosterone is the principal sex hormone men produce, it is also produced by women. It is not widely used on its own in the treatment of problems women have but is particularly useful in restoring lost sexual drive.

Oestrogens

When we talk of hormone replacement therapy after the menopause, it is usually oestrogen replacement that is meant. Two main sorts of oestrogen are used – natural and synthetic oestrogens. The natural oestrogens are usually collected from animals and are then purified. The main source is pregnant mares (hence the name of the commonest preparation, Premarin, from pregnant mare urine). These natural oestrogens have some advantages over other treatments as they have been used for many decades and a great deal is known about them. They seem to cause little in the way of side effects. Critics say that the reason for this is probably that they are not particularly powerful.

Synthetic oestrogens

Synthetic oestrogens have been used for many years. The earliest, no longer used in medicine, were derivatives of coal tar and followed from the explosion in chemistry that began in the early part of this century. The most famous of these was diethyl-stilboestrol, which is now rarely used. Since those days there have been dramatic changes in the pharmaceutical industry, and synthetic oestrogens are the basis of oral contraceptives. This means two things – they are now widely and readily available and the vast amount of research that the pill has generated means that synthetic oestrogens are better understood now than almost any other drug.

Differences between synthetic and natural oestrogens

The most important difference is one of potency. Synthetic oestrogens are designed to be much more powerful than natural hormones, which means that lower doses can be given and that there are fewer harmful side effects.

Problems with synthetic hormones

Synthetic hormones have some problems of their own. The body produces antibodies to these hormones, and these antibodies may be responsible for some of the damage to blood vessels. Oestrogens in general, and particularly synthetic oestrogens, cause an increase in blood pressure and this in turn leads to heart disease. Lots of studies have shown the links between long term use of synthetic steroids in high doses and heart and blood vessel disease.

Overgrowth of the endometrium

There is one other important effect of all oestrogens. They make the endometrium (the lining of the womb) grow. There is nothing very startling about this – it is one of their normal functions. But oestrogens given on their own and for a long time lead to a considerable overgrowth of the endometrium and there is the possibility that this may develop into a cancer. Oestrogens themselves do not cause cancer but perhaps by making the endometrium overgrow they make it more vulnerable to whatever it is that does cause cancer. At one time preventing this overgrowth of endometrium was done simply by giving oestrogens for three weeks at a time, then stopping them and allowing the woman to have a period. But most experts believe this is not enough and a much more satisfactory way of preventing overgrowth is to give additional progestogens. When these progestogens are stopped each month a period happens and when they are restarted they prevent the overgrowth of the endometrium. Taking progestogens leads to a return of periods, however, and also the premenstrual syndrome, but it does mean that there is no overgrowth of the endometrium because every month this is shed. Progestogens are not taken every day, but only for 10 to 14 days in each month.

A somewhat drastic answer

Because progestogens themselves have some side effects it has been suggested that one way to give oestrogen hormone replacement therapy without having to worry about the effect of the drug on the endometrium is to recommend that the woman receiving the treatment has a hysterectomy first. At least then she need never worry about cancerous changes occurring, or periods, or the effects of progestogens.

Progestogens

Progestogens are drugs broken down in the body to give an effect rather similar to that of progesterone. There are several different types available but all have similar effects. Because they are only used to prevent abnormal growth of the endometrium, there is little point in women who have had a hysterectomy taking them. There are theoretical benefits in taking them to prevent osteoporosis but these possible advantages do not outweigh their potential, harmful side effects.

Not given alone as hormone replacement

Because some progestogens are broken down in the body to give oestrogens, a rather naive belief arose that by giving progestogens that broke down into oestrogens, women could receive all the benefits of oestrogens without any of the dangers. Few people believe this any more. Progestogens are no longer given as hormone replacement in their own right but are used as supplements to oestrogens.

Testosterone

Testosterone alone is rarely given. It tends to be reserved for treating women who have lost their libido (their sexual drive). Loss of libido may be a hormonal problem, a psychological problem, or a response to social changes but it often originates in physical problems such as a dry vagina. Few specialists would give testosterone immediately to a woman who was worried about a lack of sexual drive or feeling. The first step in trying to help someone with such a problem is to talk the problem over and try to understand how it began. If it is the result of painful intercourse, then that physical cause should be treated first. When the physical problem has been cured – for example by replacing oestrogens to allow the vagina to function in the way it was designed – and careful counselling makes it seem that the problem is one of a loss of sexual desire in general rather than a loss of desire for the present partner, then using testosterone supplements can reverse the problem.

Effects of testosterone

The use or over use of testosterone can be dangerous. Because it is a male hormone it can cause changes in women that are sometimes permanent. Women who take testosterone do not grow beards and moustaches but they may notice an increase in facial hair and the development of acne. Very occasionally their voice deepens and although this may do no more than change its tone slightly, this can be catastrophic for someone who earns her living through her voice, such as a singer.

Giving hormones as tablets

Swallowing tablets is the most obvious way of giving medical treatment but there are some disadvantages. Pure, natural sex hormones are poorly absorbed when swallowed and this causes a problem for people who need to take them. Either the hormones must be changed to make them work when swallowed or they must be given by another route. In societies such as Britain which are pill-oriented and where both men and women prefer to take treatment as tablets rather than using any other way of getting drugs into the body, this means that the only sensible solution is for the hormones to be changed chemically into synthetic steroids. The most noted examples of this are the oral contraceptives.

Advantages of tablets

The advantages of tablets are obvious. Women have some say over the treatment because they can decide whether or not to swallow the pills, and tablets are cheap and easy to prepare. Most women have taken oral contraceptive pills at some stage of their lives and so the transition from one type of pill to another is easy. In fact, for many women the transition is rapid, they go from birth control pills to oestrogen replacement pills within a couple of years. This is not necessarily sensible, however. The birth control pill contains about six times as much oestrogen as a woman in the climacteric years needs, which means that if the transition is begun too early there is a risk of pregnancy and if it is left for too long the woman receives an overdose of hormones for the last few years she takes the contraceptive pill. This might not be harmful but is certainly unnecessary.

Disadvantages

There is one obvious disadvantage to taking tablets. For some women, taking a pill every day means 'I am ill; I need treatment'. The menopause is not a disease and so taking oestrogen replacement in a way that makes it seem as if it is a disease is counterproductive.

Another disadvantage of oral treatment is that any steroids swallowed are absorbed through the intestine and go from there to the liver, where they are passed back through the bile ducts and into the intestine again. They are then reabsorbed a second time, and this effect means that some steroid is lost without being used, and that the liver carries a disproportionate load of any side effects.

For those who do not take oral contraceptives there are two types of oral treatment: those using natural and those using synthetic oestrogens. Both of these preparations can be linked with progestogens, either in the same tablet or as separate tablets in the same course of treatment. Oral contraceptives all use synthetic steroids.

Other options

All other ways of getting hormones into the body avoid them entering the stomach and intestine, which means they are considered by many experts a much safer way of giving some drugs. Anything taken by mouth needs to go through the intestine to be absorbed, and from there the bloodstream takes it directly to the liver. The liver breaks down many of the drugs and chemicals that pass through it. This is sometimes useful (it can change inactive substances into active drugs) but it also creates difficulties because some of the byproducts of this change are themselves active as drugs, occasionally in a harmful and often in an unpredictable way. Also, the activity of the liver means that much of the dose of drug given is wasted. It is broken down before it gets a chance to act on the rest of the body, and the effect of the drug on the liver itself can be harmful. Some people believe that many of the harmful effects of synthetic steroids come from their damage to the liver as well as the changes in the body that they make the liver produce. All of this has made the pharmaceutical industry look for other ways of delivering hormones to the body.

Vaginal creams

Many of the unpleasant signs of the climacteric become obvious through the vagina. As the vaginal lining shrinks it becomes less resistant to infection and damage, intercourse becomes less pleasurable, and the vulva (the outer lips of the vagina) becomes dry, itchy, and often tender. Most of these troubles can be reversed with oestrogens, and for years treatment with oestrogen cream was recommended. There is an obvious logic in rubbing cream onto an affected part, and the cream also acts as a lubricant for intercourse.

For many years doctors could also kid themselves and their patients that this was not the same as giving hormones by mouth because the hormones in the cream were not absorbed by the body. Unfortunately this is not true. The lining of the vagina is very good at absorbing drugs, and giving oestrogen cream leads to much of the hormone in the cream getting into the rest of the body.

Problems with vaginal creams

This is not necessarily a bad thing, but the difficulty with relying on it as a way of treating oestrogen deficiency is that it means the woman is not getting a measured amount of hormone; she is receiving whatever hormone there is in the unmeasured portion of cream she applies to the vagina or vulva. This makes the endometrium grow, and normally oestrogens are given with progestogens to stop this. They should be given when oestrogen cream is being used but they rarely are.

Effect on the partner

There is one other unusual problem that occurs with vaginal oestrogen creams. They affect men. Like the vagina the skin of the penis is a good way of absorbing hormones, and some men who have regular intercourse with a partner who uses oestrogen cream suffer ill effects. This is principally the development of breasts, but some other oestrogen effects have been noted.

There are some advantages

Despite this, oestrogen creams are a good way of providing missing hormones. They are cheap to produce, do not affect the liver, and they make a contribution to the missing oestrogens for the rest of the body. They are of particular benefit for the vagina, vulva, and the urethra (the opening through which urine passes), because they have a good effect on the tissues they are rubbed in to.

Injections

Injecting the missing hormones is an obvious way of bypassing the effect of the intestine and the liver. It also makes sure that the hormone gets right into the body, in a carefully measured amount.

Disadvantages

There are obvious disadvantages. Not everybody likes injections, although for some cultures they symbolise a more powerful form of treatment. The biggest disadvantage, however, is that any natural hormone injected will be rapidly used and then broken down by the body. Diabetics get over this by injecting themselves with insulin a couple of times a day. This is hardly sensible as a treatment for women suffering the symptoms of the climacteric. So to get round this the injections used are of synthetic hormones that are broken down slowly by the body, and are often injected in a fairly thick or oily solution so that they are absorbed slowly from the injection site.

Wax pellets

Using pellets of wax is really an extension of the idea of injecting hormones in an oily solution to allow them to be absorbed slowly from the body. The hormones are mixed in wax pellets which are injected under the skin in a minor surgical procedure that takes a few minutes and needs no anaesthetic. They dissolve slowly and release the hormones gradually. Because they are larger and more solid than oily injections they are more difficult to inject under the skin, but they also last a lot longer – most for at least six months and often a year. They can contain oestrogen or testosterone and because they are broken down so slowly, natural hormones rather than synthetic ones are used. It is said that another advantage they have over injections is that if a woman changes her mind after they have been implanted, a small surgical procedure can be carried out to remove them. In practice, however, this is not really feasible and rarely works.

Silastic implants

Silastic implants are not yet available for the management of the climacteric, but when (and if) they become available they may be the ultimate answer. The hormone is contained in a silastic (a kind of plastic made of silicone) tube, which is injected under the skin. The cylinder lasts more or less for ever, and so can easily be removed if the woman concerned wants it to be. The hormone inside the cylinder leaks out through the silastic lining at a steady, constant rate, and so the hormone levels in the blood are constant, rather than swinging up and down daily the way they do when tablets are taken. There is enough hormone in the silastic implants currently being tried to last for at least seven years, although at present they are only being used to deliver contraceptive hormones.

Hormones are injected under the skin and released gradually.

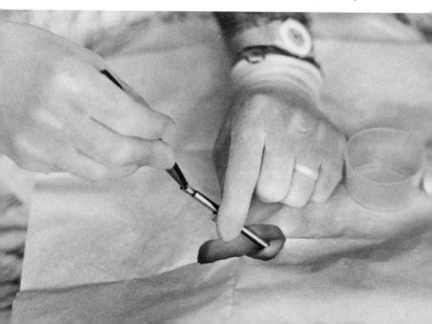

Sticking plasters

The skin is a good portal of entry for hormones. The vaginal lining is particularly good, but all skin allows hormones through, and after being absorbed through the skin the hormone goes directly into the blood stream to be carried to the rest of the body.

One problem with taking hormones through the skin is ensuring that the right dose is administered. Hormone-loaded skin patches are one solution. They are simply small sticky patches which look rather like a first aid dressing but with a solution of hormones in alcohol instead of the central gauze patch. Each patch has enough oestrogen to last for three days, and can be stuck anywhere over the body, although women are encouraged to place them somewhere between the waist and the knees. Each plaster has a measured amount of hormone, which is absorbed over the next few days, after which the woman concerned simply swops it for another. The patches are waterproof, so will last through bathing and swimming, and are of a transparent material which makes them relatively inconspicuous.

At present, only oestrogen patches are available.

Vaginal tablets (pessaries)

Vaginal tablets are called pessaries in Britain and vaginal suppositories in the USA. They have been used as a means of giving hormones to women for many years and both oestrogens and progestogens can be given this way.

For some years pessaries of progesterone have been used by doctors to treat women with some of the symptoms of the premenstrual syndrome. This syndrome is thought to be related to imbalances between the levels of oestrogen and progesterone hormones, and the hope is that by giving large amounts of additional progesterone the imbalance can be corrected. The experience gained with this means that adapting the pessaries to contain oestrogen is fairly simple.

Initially these pessaries were recommended as a means of giving oestrogens, again with the hope that they would act locally with no effects on the rest of the body. Just as the oestrogen in hormone cream is absorbed into the bloodstream, so is the oestrogen here, although there is a new pessary now available on the British market which is much less well absorbed. This will make it particularly suitable for women who have a problem in the genital area, but who cannot, or do not want to, take oestrogens into the rest of their body.

Rectal tablets (suppositories)

The lining of the rectum is a good entry for many drugs and hormones into the body. The British are rather reluctant to take medicines in this way, however, and so there are no hormone-loaded preparations on the United Kingdom market. They are available in other countries.

Vaginal rings

The vagina is a good way of absorbing medicines, but it is difficult to keep the dose there. Oestrogen hormone replacement therapy is a long term treatment and many women find it inconvenient to remember to take a tablet or put cream into the vagina every day. In addition, using any medicine every day leads to peaks and troughs of those medicines in the bloodstream. Much effort has gone into trying to develop ways of giving drugs for a long period of time in such a way that the levels are constant and people cannot forget to take their next dose.

Advantages

Vaginal rings are one such approach. They are already being widely used in parts of Europe, especially Scandinavia, and the United States of America for contraception, and are now being promoted as a means of providing oestrogens, with or without progestogens. They are simple. Each device is a ring of silastic shaped like a quoit, about 60 mm (2.75 in) across and up to 10 mm thick. The device is hollow, and filled with the hormone that is wanted. The woman puts it into the vagina, and leaves it there. There is usually enough hormone to last for six months, and the device needs no additional care. If necessary, it can be removed easily enough for washing or if it gets uncomfortable. It does not interfere with intercourse any more than a diaphragm does. Because it can be made to carry both oestrogens and progestogens this system can provide sufficient hormone replacement therapy for women who still have a uterus, as well as those who have had a hysterectomy. The oestrogen in vaginal hormone rings has an effect over the whole body, but there is a particular benefit to the genital area.

Not yet in use here

Rings are not yet being used in Britain; like many European ideas they seem to be waiting for 1992 before being offered for use here. Using progestogens in the ring has one disadvantage: part of their benefit comes from being stopped regularly, and if the same ring has both hormones, then it is difficult to arrange for the oestrogen to continue whilst the progestogens stop.

Skin cream

Mention has already been made of the effectiveness of the skin in absorbing drugs and hormones. Hormone skin cream is another way of exploiting this. These skin creams need to be rubbed into the skin every day, from where they are absorbed. Again, they bypass the liver, which means that lower doses are needed, and some harmful effects avoided.

Benefits of hormone treatment

There are definite benefits to oestrogen hormone replacement therapy. There are some conditions that can be helped only with oestrogens. There are also more intangible benefits. In the end, the importance that you place on each will decide whether you feel oestrogens are a good idea for you or not.

Treating hot flushes

The first and for some the most important use of oestrogens is in the treatment of hot flushes. There is no other form of

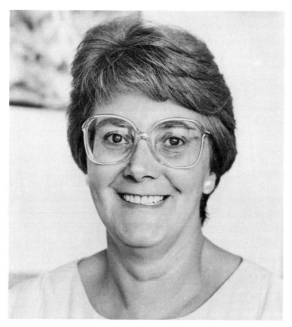

medication that is as effective as oestrogens in relieving them. For most women hot flushes are an inconvenience, a bother, that will eventually disappear. For others they are much more serious, and they will persist for up to five years. Taking oestrogens will relieve them, and if you are unhappy about taking hormones, then you do not need to take them for more than a few months. At the end of that time, stop the tablets. You will either be cured, or you won't. If the flushes recur immediately you stop the oestrogens, then start taking them again.

Vaginal problems

Rather longer term is the use of oestrogens to treat or prevent the vaginal effects of the climacteric. Again, this is something about which only you can decide but there is no doubt that oestrogens make the lining of the vagina stronger, less tender, and more able to respond to sexual stimulus. The lubrication that women produce when they are becoming aroused is not produced by glands but by changes in blood flow through the vagina. One of the first symptoms of the climacteric is changes in blood flow, and the control of small blood vessels, which shows itself in the skin as the hot flush. This is successfully treated with oestrogens and giving oestrogens will help restore lubrication.

Osteoporosis and heart disease

After those short term benefits come the longer term ones. The controversy over them is beginning to be resolved. Oestrogens prevent osteoporosis and seem to prevent heart disease. Both of these are important causes of death and disability. But for both to be treated with any success oestrogens are needed for many years, starting within three years of the last period. For the prevention of both problems oestrogens alone are not sufficient – heart disease prevention also depends on stopping smoking, improving diet, and getting more exercise. Preventing osteoporosis needs oestrogens, exercise, and a good diet.

Effects on the breasts

There are three more speculative reasons for taking oestrogens. Femininity is hard to define, but many women who take oestrogens say that they feel more feminine, and less neutered. There is certainly a beneficial effect on breast tissue, and the gradual wasting away of the breasts after the menopause is slowed with oestrogens. Femininity is not only breasts however, it is much more, and oestrogens seem to improve the whole being.

Skin

Similarly, skin changes occur throughout life, but the menopause is associated with a rapid increase in skin ageing. It is not easy to tell the effects of oestrogen loss from those of getting old, but women who take oestrogen get an increase in skin thickness, or at least the gradual thinning and loss of collagen (the connective tissue that holds skin together) is prevented.

Sexuality

There is also an effect of oestrogen on sexuality. Oestrogens are important for the reflexes that lubricate the vagina and contribute to sexual satisfaction. When the vagina is dry and painful, sexual happiness is impaired. Testosterone can improve loss of sexual desire. All of these are difficult to measure.

Risks of hormone treatment

In the doses that are used, oestrogens and progestogens are fairly safe but there are three principal dangers – breast cancer, endometrial cancer, and heart disease.

Breast cancer

The breasts are sensitive to hormones. There is much evidence that breast cancer is linked to hormonal change and giving oestrogens to women at a time when the breast is undergoing change can be potentially harmful. The evidence is beginning to emerge that menopausal oestrogen replacement therapy can make breast cancer more likely to develop. This is covered in the next chapter.

Endometrial cancer

Oestrogens make the endometrium grow, and if this growth becomes disorganised cancer can develop. This can be prevented by adding progestogens, however, and fear of cancer of the endometrium should never inhibit oestrogen treatment.

Heart disease from added progestogens

Progestogens are not entirely risk-free. They may make heart disease more likely to occur, and so trying to prevent endometrial cancer may put women at risk of heart disease from the progestogens. If there is such a risk it is minimal.

For how long should treatment continue?

This is your decision. If you want relief from hot flushes, then oestrogens for a year are probably all you need. If you want protection from heart disease and osteoporosis, then change your diet and your exercise habits, stop smoking, and take oestrogens for 10 years. If you want to preserve 'femininity', then perhaps oestrogens for the rest of your life is what you want.

Who should not take hormones?

On medical grounds there are probably very few women who should not take oestrogens. Untreated cancer of the endometrium or breast should disqualify anyone from taking hormones, but what about those women who have been treated? For many people quality of life is as important as quantity, and if you feel that the real risks of an earlier death outweigh those of an improved life through an absence of hot flushes or vaginal dryness, then the choice must be yours.

The decision is yours

In the end you must decide for yourself. Oestrogen hormone replacement therapy may improve the quality of your life. There is good evidence that for most women it will improve the quantity of life by preventing premature death from heart disease and perhaps by preventing premature death from the complications of a broken hip. But only you can decide whether or not those benefits outweigh the small, but real risk of death from cancer of the breast. Cancer of the endometrium should not happen in women who take oestrogens because the risk is well recognised and understood, and the use of added progestogens should remove it. In the next chapter we shall take a closer look at cancer.

9 Cancer

People seem to be more afraid of cancer than any other disease. Irrational fears about their ability to cause cancer have led to useful chemicals being abandoned, although ironically natural substances known to be harmful are usually left alone. Many governments act irrationally over cancer and screening for it. Cancer is an unpleasant disease, and treatments of many forms are no more successful now than was the case 40 years ago.

Some common factors in cancers

Different cancers have different causes, but they nearly all have a few things in common. They are more likely to occur in older people, and the longer you live the more likely you are to get one. They are also more likely to happen to people who live in more affluent societies, perhaps because they live longer. And when cancers can be prevented there is often no great desire to prevent them.

What are the facts?

Yet many cancers are preventable, and even when all are added together the unpreventable cancers are not particularly important as causes of death in Britain. But fear of cancer, especially the cancers caused by hormones, is real and common. What are the facts?

Cancers in British women

For many years the commonest cause of cancer death in British women was breast cancer, which is rare in Third World countries. It has now been overtaken by lung cancer, but this is probably because cigarette consumption is rising rather than because breast cancer is becoming less common. Cancer of the cervix, endometrium, and ovary are much less common than breast cancer. There are some cancers that are linked to hormones, and these are especially important to women contemplating hormone treatment. These will be discussed individually.

Breast cancer

Breast cancer is common and important. It is no longer the commonest cancer that affects British women, but is one of the most feared, because of the mutilation it leads to. The chances of being cured after a diagnosis of breast cancer are pretty much the same now as they were 50 years ago. It is one of the first cancers where a hormonal link was suspected, but proof of that link is as elusive as ever. So what is known about breast cancer?

Breast cancer mainly occurs in women but when it does occur in men it often follows oestrogen hormone treatment. It occurs in women who have had a lot of exposure to hormones, and so is common amongst women who have other cancers, such as from the ovary, that produce additional hormones. It also occurs among women who received high doses of diethyl-stilboestrol in early pregnancy. But all of these are minor causes of breast cancer, and much more important are things over which few women have any control, or if they do, by the time they reach the menopause it is too late to change them.

Factors in breast cancer

Factors include your age when you had your first period, the regularity of your periods in the first few years after they started, and the age at which your first baby was born. Women who are infertile because they have not ovulated are also at an increased risk of breast cancer. All of these factors suggest that hormonal influences on the breast at particularly vulnerable times can lead to cancer developing many years later. Taking additional hormones, perhaps for years on end, does not seem to have nearly the same effect. This explains why women who take oral contraceptive pills for many years do not seem to develop breast cancer as a result (and there is even a possibility that the pill is protective, but most experts discount this), but additional hormones at a vulnerable time such as pregnancy are harmful.

X-ray of the breast: mammogram.

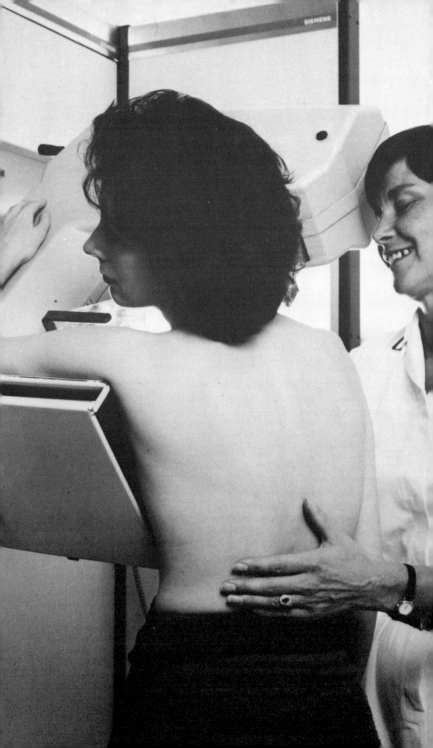

Is the menopause a vulnerable time?

No one is sure yet whether the menopause is a vulnerable time. Breast cancer is more common in women who have passed the menopause and this continually rising incidence makes analysis of the figures difficult. Women who live longer are much more likely to develop breast cancer than those who die young, which is another confounding factor.

Important points

Oestrogens are the main hormones that act on breast tissue to make it grow. Giving women drugs that act against oestrogen to prevent it from having an effect slows down the growth of many breast cancers, as does removing many of the sources of oestrogens from a woman – for example by removing her ovaries.

What about giving oestrogens to women after their own oestrogen production has stopped? There have been dozens of attempts at studying this, which itself suggests there is no clear and easy answer. There is perhaps a slight increase in the risk of breast cancer from taking oestrogen replacement, although some studies suggest that if progestogens are added to the treatment programme the risk is reduced again. And breast cancer becomes less likely for women who take both oestrogens and progestogens than it is for women who take no hormones.

A small risk

Overall, there may be a tiny added risk of breast cancer in women who take oestrogen hormone replacement. This means that some doctors suggest that women who have, or have recently had treatment for breast cancer, do not take additional oestrogens. This is still debatable so you should discuss it with your doctor. If flushes or fears of osteoporosis are making your life a misery, then the small risk of oestrogen treatment may be outweighed by the potential benefits.

Endometrial cancer

At least for this cancer there is little argument about the evidence. Giving oestrogens is responsible for making the endometrium grow and stopping giving progesterone for allowing it to be shed.

In the early days of oestrogen hormone replacement treatment not enough attention was paid to this. Now most women who have oestrogens take additional progestogens, usually for the same length of time that their bodies would produce progesterone during a normal ovulatory cycle. This means that they take progestogens for about two weeks, then stop them, which will precipitate a period if there is any endometrium produced by the oestrogens.

Ovarian cancer

Ovarian cancer becomes more common as women age, and is prevented in younger women by taking oestrogen-containing oral contraceptives. There is no reason to believe that giving oestrogens will cause this cancer to develop in women who have passed the menopause. But at the same time the dose of oestrogen that is given for hormone replacement treatment is probably too small to prevent ovarian cancer developing. Perhaps regular examinations in a clinic will detect any cancer that develops early but even that is a small hope.

Cervical cancer

Cancer of the cervix has been talked about more than almost any other female cancer, except perhaps cancer of the breast. It has probably been the subject of more news bulletins and parliamentary discussion than any other. Because it has a recognisable early stage that can be detected through cervical smears, screening for it has become almost a marker for the concern that health authorities have for women's health problems.

No link with hormone treatment

First, the good news. There is no link between taking any form of hormonal replacement therapy and cancer of the cervix. There are, however, very strong links between cigarette smoking, your partner's occupation, and you and your partner's sexual experiences and cancer of the cervix.

Have regular check ups

What is important is the fact that cancer of the cervix becomes more common in women who are in the years of the climacteric. But because most doctors perform a cervical smear before they discuss hormone replacement treatment any cancer or precancer of the cervix will be detected early. It is possible that by keeping the genital tract healthy, hormone treatment will make it easier for a cancer to be detected in the first place. Certainly, regular visits to a clinic will also help.

If you have had cancer of the cervix, or even simply abnormal smears, there is no reason at all for you not to take oestrogens.

Should women who have had cancer take oestrogens?

Economists who study the health service talk about the quality of life and ways of trying to get the most improvement in it for the greatest number of people. For many potential treatments they try and weigh the balance between quality and quantity of life, and perhaps the only thing they agree on is that it is extremely difficult to do. There is no doubt that for most women oestrogens increase both the quality and quantity of life but for those who have had cancers, the equation is more difficult to balance.

No problem with most cancers

Cancer of the ovary, cervix, and other parts of the body should not influence your decision at all. If you have had the skin cancer, malignant melanoma, talk things over with the specialist looking after you. This is because some of these cancers are oestrogen-sensitive – they respond to additional oestrogens by growing more wildly.

More difficult decisions

The difficulties come with cancer of the breast and cancer of the endometrium. Both of these are sensitive to hormones, and both grow under the influence of oestrogen. Cancer of the endometrium will often shrink if progestogens are given but

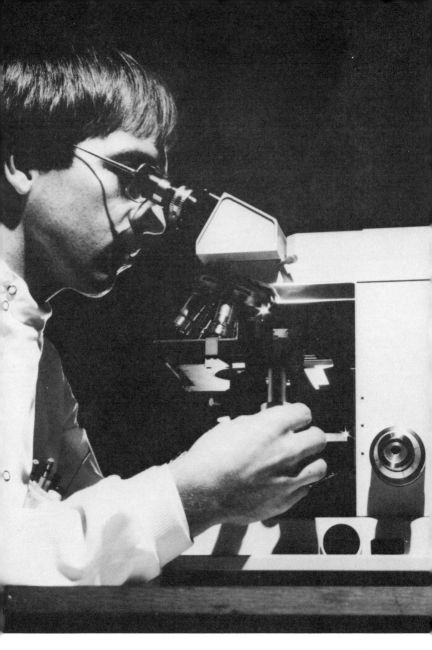

Cancer of the cervix can be detected at an early stage by cervical smears screening.

progestogens do not seem to affect most breast cancers. Endometrial cancer is usually treated surgically, and once it has been treated there is no reason not to start, or restart oestrogens, if that is what you want. If you have had breast cancer the situation is more complex. If your breast cancer was oestrogen sensitive, or you do not know whether or not it was, then it may not be a good idea to take oestrogens – but the decision must be yours. If the cancer was not oestrogen sensitive, there is probably no reason not to take oestrogens. Talk it over with your doctor.

10 Where do you go from here?

Any book that lists the possible problems women face at the menopause probably ends up making everything about it seem unpleasant, which is not true. The menopause can be a very positive time, when you can begin to plan for the rest of your life. But you do need to plan. You need to plan for the exercise you need to keep your heart and bones healthy. You need to plan the way your life and career is going to develop over the next few years. And you need to discuss the question of hormone replacement treatment with your doctor.

Menopause clinics

If you don't especially want to see your family doctor, you can get some help from family planning clinics, well woman clinics, or menopause clinics. There are special menopause clinics in many parts of the country. When you get there the first thing to happen will be for someone to sit down with you and talk to you about the problems you may have had and your hopes for the future.

What will happen?

If you decide to start hormone replacement treatment, and the decision is yours, then most doctors will examine you, and take a cervical smear if you are due for one (which is often why it is best to see your own doctor first; he or she will know from your records if you are due one). Your blood pressure will be checked, you will be weighed, blood samples may be taken so that your levels of follicle stimulating hormone can be measured, and then an appropriate oestrogen preparation, perhaps with additional progestogens, will be prescribed. The follicle stimulating hormone level is measured because if it is raised it confirms the presence of the climacteric, and if it falls in response to giving oestrogens it suggests that treatment is working.

Keeping an eye on you

Most clinics and GPs will want to see you again every six months or so just to make sure there are no problems developing. They will always leave the door open for you to come back sooner, however, if anything unforeseen occurs.

Self help

The menopause is a stage of life – it is not a disease or disorder, although some of its 'symptoms' can cause problems and may need medical help. The most important person in seeing you through all these changes is yourself. Although the menopause marks the end of your reproductive life it most certainly does not mean that your productive life is over. In fact, many women really come into their own when they are in their 50s. It is essential, however, to maintain your confidence and your sense of self esteem at a time when so many social, emotional, and bodily changes are taking place and when there seems to be a widening gap between what you would like to achieve and what is possible. Look after yourself physically and emotionally. Make plans, develop new interests, and enjoy yourself. Life after 50 can be fun.

Index